Macrobiotic Guidebook For Living

AND OTHER ESSAYS

Macrobiotic Guidebook For Living

·AND OTHER ESSAYS·

by George Ohsawa

Translated by Herman Aihara

Edited by Paula Markham

George Ohsawa Macrobiotic Foundation
Oroville, California

First publication in Japanese - 1947

First English edition - © 1967
   Ohsawa Foundation, Los Angeles, California

Revised English edition - © 1985
   George Ohsawa Macrobiotic Foundation
   1511 Robinson Street, Oroville, California 95965

ISBN No. 0-918860-41-5

Typeset in 10 point Century Expanded
Typesetting by Sylvia Zuck, G.O.M.F. staff
Layout by Susan Reid
Cover design by John Clarke, New York City
Printing by Delta Lithograph Company, Van Nuys, California

Acknowledgments

The efforts of many people have gone into the realization of this book. Thanks to Lou Oles and Shayne Oles Suehle for their editing of the 1967 edition of the *Guidebook*; to Tom Goldwasser, Susan Jacobowitz, and Maya Edwards for their work on the *Practical Guide to Far Eastern Macrobiotic Medicine* from which several essays have been taken; to John Clarke for cover design; and to Susan Reid, Sylvia Zuck, Paula Markham, and all the G.O.M.F. staff who have helped bring this book to its present form. Unending thanks to George and Lima Ohsawa.

Herman Aihara

Editor's Note

The *Macrobiotic Guidebook for Living* was originally published in 1947 in Japan, where it was very successful. It was translated into English by Herman Aihara and published in 1967 by the Ohsawa Foundation in Los Angeles, California.

In the present edition, the text of the *Guidebook* has been rearranged slightly for clarity. Additional material on child care, which was printed in the 1967 edition as a separate essay, has been incorporated in the text.

The first five essays in the *Essays* section are reprinted from *Practical Guide to Far Eastern Macrobiotic Medicine* (G.O.M.F. Press, 1973). "Your Biography Before Birth" appeared as a separate essay in the 1967 edition of the *Guidebook*. "The Seven Stages of Judgment" is reprinted from *The Book of Judgment* (G.O.M.F. Press, 1980). "The Order of the Universe and the Unique Principle" is reprinted from *Atomic Age and the Philosophy of the Far East* (G.O.M.F. Press, 1977).

P.M.

CONTENTS

Macrobiotic Guidebook for Living

Other Essays

Foreword to the Original Edition

I have suffered misgivings in calling this volume *The Macrobiotic Guidebook for Living* since I have no qualifications as a teacher of morals, much less the ambition to be one. My biggest desire is to give of my years of experience in dealing with a fundamental relationship — the one that exists between food and life.

As you read you will surely conclude, and with good reason, that I have been a gourmand all my life! I have been so big an eater that I have surprised and frightened myself more than once.

I thus know the dangers inherent in eating through personal experience. What could be a more open confession of my struggles with the problem of over-eating than my activity as a teacher of diet?

My big appetite would surely have brought me to an early, miserable death had I not been engaged in an unending search for the secret of food. It was most fortunate that near the end, when I was almost dead, I found macrobiotics.

George Ohsawa
Japan, 1947

Introduction

I believe that we cannot achieve anything important if we do not have a strong stomach. If we cannot eat all things, we are unhappy. As the result of understanding macrobiotics, I can now maintain health and happiness while eating anything I desire. My writing is the condensation of such understanding and experience.

I have met so many unhappy people in my life — they consult me every day. I can sympathize with them since I myself was once such a person. After hearing about my experiences, they imitate the way of living I have evolved and soon overcome their difficulties. This is what has made me more and more confident in the macrobiotic way of life.

During one of my seminars I visually diagnosed an old woman who sat in front of me. It was very obvious to me that she had been separated from her husband and I told her so. "Yes, I have been alone thirty years," she replied, startled. For a long time she had been eating the things that could cause such separation — sugar, fruit, or generally yin (expansive) food — and it showed in her physical make-up. She was impotent, could not conceive, and had developed a hatred for men which caused them to avoid her instinctively. Her life had long been a miserable one.

Our faces mirror two things: 1) the food eaten by our mothers from the time of conception; and 2) what we have eaten since birth.

Mr. Nanboku Mizuno, an authority on the diagnosis of an individual's past and future, fate, and character, was asked how one could reach his level of understanding and possess his secret. "Study everyday food," was his answer. Mizuno, a masseur in a Turkish bath, talked with countless numbers of people every day during his work. He endlessly engaged in the small talk that covered an individual's constitution, parentage, and place of birth. After many years of this kind of experience, he worked out the relationship between facial characteristics, bone structure, fate, character, and food.

Like Nanboku, I have learned much from observing people. Their constitutions and faces tell me what their daily eating has been. At times, this is troublesome because when I see an individual, I see *food.* Some people look like fruit or sugar, others look like milk, eggs, steak, or ham! And as soon as I see what their daily food in the past has been, I can picture their everyday life at the present — their families, friendships, financial problems, thoughts, character and mentality. I can see what their sickness is, where it is, and when it began. I can tell when and how a woman's menstruation occurs and what the condition of her ovaries is. In short, I can see whether the person before me is happy or unhappy.

Recently I met a man who had come to Japan to preach religion. Noting his eyebrows, I foresaw misfortune in his future. His inability to give up eating the one particular bad food prohibited by his religion was very obvious. I realized he was a hypocrite. Nevertheless, fifty people listened to him lecture and were much moved; I myself learned very much from him. And yet I wondered about his future.

Only yesterday I attended a group meeting of prominent people in the field of economics where we discussed him. It was revealed that my foreign friend had been purged from his religious organization; he was openly called a liar. This confirmed my diagnosis of him on the basis of food.

Good luck or bad, happiness or unhappiness, longevity or early death, wisdom or stupidity, beauty or ugliness, goodness or badness — all are determined by eating. When we understand this fully, we see that men are neither good nor bad; they are only the products of good or bad eating.

The Macrobiotic Guidebook for Living is devoted to our destiny in life; our happiness or unhappiness as based on food. It thus differs widely from the sort of guidance for life offered in the writings of many great men.

George Ohsawa

Chapter 1

Love

Food and the phenomena of life are very closely related; where there is no food, there are no phenomena of life. Growth, size, strength, wisdom, ignorance, ideas, attitudes, activities, the rise and fall of race and nation — all are affected. They are determined and controlled by what we eat and drink. Love and marriage, the fundamentals of social living, are no exceptions to this rule.

It is common knowledge that there are no bigger drives in our lives than sexual desire and hunger for food. There has been much discussion as to which is more primary. Even those who have managed to detach themselves from sexual desire find that the need for nourishment is with them always. Hunger is the most powerful motivation for man. If we do not eat for a long enough period of time, we die. The profound influence of hunger is felt as long as we live. Whoever wants to realize the full strength of his hunger has only to fast for a few days.

I do not mean to play down the strength of sexual desire; history is witness to the intensity of its force. It has undone heroes and brought emperors to the level of the common man. It has even given birth to the saying, "Behind every crime is a woman."

On the simplest level, we are alive because of our appetite for food. If we are at all thankful for that life, we are expressing our gratitude for the hunger that is its driving force. He who has a healthy appetite can enjoy the simplest meal. Who can afford to be without it?

I believe that any concept of the universe that claims to be the true way for man, the path that leads to complete fulfillment, must teach a practical method for achieving the following goals:

1. the hunger without which individual life ceases to exist, and
2. the sexual love that underlies all social living — that of race, nation, and all humanity.

This is macrobiotics.

* * *

Within the range of human desire, craving for food appears very early — the first day after birth. When we hear a baby cry for its mother's milk and then see it at the breast, we are witnessing the miraculous power of the will to live.

At the age of seven or eight, a child shows signs of intellectual desire — the need to know. At the same time, an awareness of the opposite sex comes into being. Around fourteen, girls commence to menstruate, while boys become manly in structure and character at about sixteen. The biological structure of a female is complete by twenty-one; she is then ready for motherhood. Boys in turn are physiologically prepared for parenthood and seek out the opposite sex as they approach twenty-four.

These are the ages of love for both male and female and are inevitable. Although the precise periods may differ slightly from one race or nation to another, they generally follow this pattern.

One thing is certain: if by the ages of twenty-one for girls and twenty-four for boys the desire for the opposite sex has not appeared, it is not only unnatural but a sign of deep illness. It is caused by eating habits that are not in accord with the orderliness of the universe. A grave dietary error has been made during the first seven years for the female or the first eight years for the male. Those who carefully observe the macrobiotic diet avoid this difficulty. They are strongly attracted sexually and know the joys of love.

* * *

It is interesting that physiological and spiritual changes occur in cycles of seven years for the female (at seven, fourteen, twenty-one, etc.) and eight years for the male (at eight, sixteen, twenty-four, etc.). Biologically speaking, the cells of the human organism are completely changed every seven years. Girls, more yang at birth than boys, are drawn to yin foods and change rapidly in accord with this biological law. Boys, more yin when born, are attracted to yang with the result that change for them is slower — every eight years. Here we see the key to the biological superiority of the female.

For example, women are mature by the age of twenty-eight (four times seven) and a strong sexual life begins for them. No wonder that these have been called the dangerous and troublesome years. At thirty-five (five times seven) they become quieter and a spiritual quality begins to show itself. At forty-two (six times seven) their spiritual life has deepened; at forty-nine (seven times seven) menstruation and sexual life cease and women become peaceful at last.

Boys mature as men at thirty-two (four times eight). At forty (five times eight) the spiritual life begins and has deepened enough by the age of forty-eight (six times eight) for them to become thinkers; steadiness becomes very apparent. A man begins harvesting the fruits of his life at fifty-six (seven times eight); at sixty-four (eight times eight) his sexual life ends and his true, peaceful life of deepest spirituality commences.

For both sexes, six times their cycle (forty-eight for men and forty-two for women) marks the dividing line between the physical and the spiritual life. From this time on, they are more and more detached from the materialistic flesh and can attain a spirituality that is peaceful and eternal; they are free.

There are those people whose lives are so divorced from the orderliness of nature that they never enter this realm; they spend all their years involved with sex and appetite and are most unfortunate.

* * *

It is one of the primordial laws of nature that yin and yang are strongly attracted to one another. In the case of male (yang) and female (yin), the attraction must be strong enough for them to be able to hold together in an enduring, happy marriage.

At the seventh year, the female begins to develop distinctly feminine characteristics and the male, distinctly masculine ones. From here on, if care is taken, girls become progressively more feminine (yin) and boys more masculine (yang). It has been traditional in many cultures, notably the Oriental ones, to separate boys and girls as much as possible from this time on. They neither sit together nor play together in schools or playgrounds and are kept somewhat apart until marriage.

The characteristics that distinguish one sex from the other are given little chance to become blurred by the familiarity that results from continuous social contact. Yin becomes more yin and yang more yang. Nurtured thus, the power to attract the opposite sex has the opportunity to grow as strong as possible. (Brothers and sisters of course are the exception to the rule of separation, since they live under the same roof and cannot avoid being together. Can this be the reason why they are sexually attracted to one another only under abnormal circumstances?)

After fourteen to eighteen years such females will have developed their full yin potential, males their full yang potential. This is particularly so if they have followed a macrobiotic way of living. Yang represents centripetal force and yin centrifugal force. So, in love, the male (yang on the surface) is aggressive, while the female (yin on the surface) is passive. This is a natural phenomenon. In fact the whole idea of love is natural — as natural as the appetite for food. It is a false idea to treat it as either divine or sinful.

The attitudes of men and women towards all things are exactly the opposite, just as yang and yin are opposed to one another. At the age of thirty-two (four times eight) a man becomes concerned with materialistic matters such as business, occupation, or position in life; he becomes a pragmatist. The woman of twenty-eight (four times seven), on the other hand, is involved with more abstract, romantic ideas; she is the romantic.

In love, man is the hunting dog in pursuit of a rabbit — oblivious of mountain, valley, or stream. He sees the game, never the surroundings; he feels the joy of the chase, never the difficulty. Woman by contrast is the rabbit — she desperately seeks a place to hide.

When a rabbit does not flee but follows or even chases the dog, the situation is no longer a natural one; she is either sick, or cruel, or both . . . a wolf in rabbit's clothing! After marriage, such a rabbit will either kill her mate by making his life miserable or take off after another dog and disappear. Whoever understands this will find success in love.

"Love is blind," noted writers like Chaucer, Shakespeare, Coleridge, and Emerson. With the appearance of love, life inevitably becomes complicated. Everything is affected when it bursts in upon us; love adds depth, beauty, and art to an existence that would be tasteless without it. There are countless stories in the literature of every country which express the many facets of this moving drama. Sometimes the power of love is so strong that we are overwhelmed and can understand neither its significance nor its meaning in our lives.

How important that so powerful an emotion be properly directed! Our life is a tragedy if we fail. And how easy it is to establish this good direction if we follow a macrobiotic way of eating!

It is interesting and amusing that in old age we find that this emotion has dwindled away like a pebble disappearing into a pool of water. That it was once so irresistible is hard to believe.

To sum up, the man who takes too many sweets in boyhood will become impotent in adolescence; too much meat will make him cruel and violent in his sexual behavior. The greatest misfortune, however, has befallen the individual who eats a combination of extreme foods (sweets, meat, dairy products, coffee, laboratory-produced foods) that eventually leave him with no sexual life at all.

Study the culture of any country — art, biography, drama, history, movies, novels, philosophy, poetry — and keep in mind eating habits. You will soon see the close connection between nourishment and love. You will understand why those who grow up macrobiotically can control their sexuality.

This is but one practical application of the yin-yang theory; the "Unique Principle" of macrobiotics.[1]

Chapter 2

Marriage

Marriage has been called the graveyard of love. I myself have seen so few happily married couples that I am inclined to agree. Since love is often only blindly emotional or instinctual, marriage usually ends in sadness and bitterness.

We all seek happiness in our lives. Yet most of us forget that married life — the well-spring from which the family grows —can and must be the factory that produces this happiness.

What makes a family happy? Mental and physical health, first of all. Macrobiotics is the most practical, easy way to fulfill this requirement. Out of my small fund of experience and knowledge I have concluded that:

1. the fundamental material for the factory of married life is food, and
2. the principle that guides us in dealing with this material and gives it order is the Unique Principle.

The Unique Principle has its basis in the orderliness of the universe in which we live. It is fundamental not only to politics, economics, and the arts, but to physics, chemistry, industry, agriculture, and commerce as well. It is the primary principle of creation, growth, and all religion.

With the Unique Principle as my basis, I have come to believe that for married life to be a source of happiness for both male and female, the following must prevail:

Physical Condition of Men

The ages most suitable for marriage are approximately twenty-four to twenty-eight. The individual's physical condition must be good from the standpoint of macrobiotics or, at the very least, he must have an understanding of this ancient wisdom. If a woman wants to choose a suitable husband, she had best test his attitude toward or reaction to it.

The easiest way to diagnose a man's condition is as follows: first, look at his ears. They are not a barometer of present health but of one's destiny or fate. If a man has been raised macrobiotically he will have large ears that lie flat against his head; the earlobes will be soft. If the lobes are exceedingly long, he will be a successful leader or very rich. There will be a happy ending to his life. A man whose ears stick out or have small lobes or no lobes at all will often suffer both physical and mental difficulties in his life. This general rule applies to Occidentals and Africans as well as Orientals. The importance of this part of the body has long been recognized throughout the world and has found expression in the widespread custom of wearing an earring. Primitive peoples have long honored those who possess the ear described above. (Note statues of Buddha and native African sculpture.)

Physical Condition of Women

Females are best suited for marriage during the years from eighteen to twenty-two, although there certainly are many women who make good wives after they have reached the age of thirty. The ear is just as important for them as it is for men. In addition, however, we must consider the eyes, nose, lips, and teeth. If a female has bad teeth, her organs are bound to be worse; to marry her can be tragic. Since she is the original source of nourishment for the children she may bear, her ability to chew — so vital for everyone — is of even greater importance. As the mothers of our sons, women must be healthier than their men. Nevertheless, please do not be worried, discouraged, or feel that all is lost if you see yourself in the above description. You can change all things through macrobiotics.

Mental Condition of Men

The most important characteristic for a man is bravery. In addition, he must also have the following traits: strength, reliability, firmness, adaptability, courage, and tolerance. Such a man wakes up early in the morning with a clear head and bright outlook. He is not a big eater of sweets nor a big drinker of alcohol.

The brave man must have a well-supported body; his feet must be surely and firmly on the ground. He wears the bottoms of his shoes evenly. If he wears the toe or heel on either side, he does not fulfill the above conditions.

Mental Condition of Women

The most important characteristics for women are self-denial, tolerance, sweetness, and punctuality — in a word, womanliness. I do not imply that a woman must be obedient. I simply mean that she *should not be stubborn.* If you are interested in changing a stubborn woman into a sweet girl, you will have a very interesting marriage.

A French poet once said, "Never hit a woman, not even with a flower." Unfortunately, the woman who merits such treatment is rare today. In Japan, they say "You must hit a woman, and with a stone if necessary." Do not marry such a woman, however. If you find the need to hit her, she will never be a good woman even if you do.

* * *

Before you marry, study your future mate's character and that of his or her parents; consider their viewpoints and family life. A strong family heritage and tradition is much more important than knowledge or education. Better that people be poor and steeped in tradition than rich and without a heritage; they are more likely to be deep and serious-minded.

If we compare life to a voyage, man is the pilot of the ship —the captain who at times must fight a raging tempest. Woman is the engineer or fireman. Her job requires tolerance, punctuality, and gentle strength.

Even if we marry with care we often end in sadness because of poor judgment. It is the combined judgment of husband and wife, working together, that goes into building a happy family. Togetherness is most important, for only through the cooperation and effort of both husband and wife can a happy family result. Epictetus said, *"Everyone is happy. If not, it is his own fault."*

The choice of raw materials is a fundamental consideration in the building of any structure; in the case of the family it consists of what we eat and drink every day. I recommend macrobiotic eating and drinking because it can lead to absolute health, and is economical as well. If you have a successful marriage but do not follow macrobiotics, you are courting disaster. If your marriage is already unsuccessful, you can change it radically for the better through macrobiotics.

Men tend to lead women mentally and theoretically; women tend to lead men physiologically. Men must try to love while women must strive to be loved; one is aggressive, the other passive.

To make one's self lovable sounds simple but in reality it is quite difficult. Many women have the idea that men have a *natural obligation* to love them, i.e., that women have the natural right to be loved. They don't consider whether or not they deserve love, nor do they make any attempt to make themselves lovable. I think this attitude is wrong for this reason: prior to the right to be loved comes the requirement that you make yourself someone to be loved. Love comes only to those who try to be loved; only a very unhappy person does not even make an attempt. The woman who tries to be loved will be happy in the end even if she marries a bad husband because the effort itself brings great happiness.

Our life looks short at times but in reality it is quite long. If after one or even five years you are tired of the chore of building a happy marriage, you are not macrobiotic.

All of us readily agree that tolerance is a virtue. Since we are human beings and not as tolerant as God, however, we find it difficult to turn the other cheek and *like* or *love* what we have come to hate. Such a high degree of understanding in our practical, everyday life is hard to achieve.

Macrobiotics can be of great help here. It teaches that bad character and behavior are only superficial; if we judge a man by them, it does not give us a true picture of the individual. They are simply the product of a long period of bad eating and poor living conditions — environment. If we understand this, we can transmute hatred into sympathy, bitterness into pity.

So . . . for a happy life, women must strive to deserve love, men must endeavor to love. Since the prerequisite for both is eating and living according to the order in nature — macrobiotics — I feel it necessary to make clear the method whereby this can be done.

Chapter 3

Family

The family has always been a primary consideration in traditional cultures. Because it is the basic building block of society, much depends upon its condition. If it is unhealthy, the nation is sick; if it is unhappy, the nation is miserable.

The creation of a healthy family is very difficult because in addition to the material, practical factors involved, there is the spiritual, intangible aspect to be considered. A strong will and a great amount of effort are required.

Man's first step toward becoming a social being was his creation of the family unit. With this, he unknowingly entered the realm of art, because the growth of a happy family is dynamic, never static. There is incessant activity, constant change, and the need for endless creativity.

I deeply admire those who have been successful at this task — a warm, bright family is the resting place of the soul, the root of life, and the spring of vitality. If our household is gloomy, sad and cold, life is so miserable; we are bound to search elsewhere for joy, pleasure, and comfort. How often have the strongest and most dependable men been forced into this position! No matter how brave a man is, if his wife is not gentle, their home will always be cold and without joy and their children will be unhappy.

William Pitt, the British politician, once said, "My success today is due solely to the efforts of my wife. She has made my home lovely and joyful, a place in which I find rest and a source for my activity." The wife of Socrates, by contrast, threw buckets of water on him while he was thinking.

Confucius, in turn, felt that "women and small-minded men are hard to communicate with."

The wife of Jinsai Ito (the Shintoist scholar who brought Chinese philosophy to Japan one hundred years ago) never bothered her husband with financial matters. During the time that he was thinking and studying, she did not disturb him even though she never knew if they would eat the next day. In spite of the fact that their life was a struggle and full of hardship, the whole family lived with hope and confidence because of her. There was happiness and joy, no matter what was lacking financially.

Whether a home is happy or not depends upon the health of its inhabitants. Emerson said, "Health is the first condition of happiness." If we are without it, we cannot achieve anything even though we have money, knowledge, good children, or a good mate. A healthy family is a happy, joyful one.

Here the importance of the mother or wife cannot be overemphasized. In her hands lies control of the life source, the well-spring of power — *the kitchen.* She must be willing to acknowledge the importance and dangers of food. She must have clarity of mind and be gentle, careful, tolerant, clever. She must know and understand macrobiotics and be capable of applying her knowledge at all times.

Some people understand macrobiotics very quickly; others take time. Scientists of repute have found it difficult to understand and apply while poor laborers have understood quickly and applied it very easily. In the field of macrobiotics, it does not matter whether you are well-educated and successful, or just a workman. All must start from the beginning.

The individual who understands macrobiotics knows and is thankful for:

    a. the wonder of living,
    b. the value of living,
    c. the joy of living,
    d. the aim or purpose of living, and
    e. that which is the greatest happiness of living.

He is always considering important things such as the value, the aim, and the joy of existence. *He is happy to be alive.*

No schooling is needed for us to be able to think about such big questions and reach valid conclusions. Formal education actually stands in the way of our considering them. There is no specially-learned method by which to deal with matters like these; all that is needed is a gentle, humble, and unassuming mind, and the answers present themselves.

Today, however, no one has the time or inclination to consider such questions even superficially. We are too busy worrying about health, security, or unpredictables like the stock market or the possibility of revolution.

But even if you are a millionaire now, you can be a beggar tomorrow morning as the result of earthquake, storm, riot, panic, theft, or betrayal.

To understand the importance of food — macrobiotics — is essential if we are not to become inextricably involved in the petty details of living. Without macrobiotics, our families and lives are miserable even if we have the good fortune to achieve high honor or position. In fact, the greater the honor or position or fortune, the greater the misery.

My belief is that an understanding of macrobiotics is *fundamental* to living; it is a study that must be undertaken by both husband and wife. Only thus can the family be joyful, bright, restful, and a prime source of energy.

First of all, the wife or mother must establish her own health; the health of her husband and children will follow. The kitchen is the pharmacy of life, and she is the pharmacist. She is the planner of culture, the director of the play. She determines whether it is tragic or joyful. Though her husband may be cruel, stubborn, or stupid, the wife who understands macrobiotics well enough can change him even if it takes three, five, ten, or twenty years. The longer it takes and the more difficulties there are to overcome, the greater the significance of her achievement. The biggest task always takes the longest time.

In this sense, the evolution of humanity depends primarily upon the judgment of women. If women only realized their own significance, if they could only see that happiness or unhappiness for all depends primarily on them, their everyday difficulties would lend a very large joy to their lives. The wife who marries a stupid husband, therefore, is that much more happy because she faces a bigger task.

If I were a woman, I would clean house with love. I would think, "How joyful, how rewarding is our life!" Whether cooking or scrubbing, polishing or dusting, I would think, "I am creating life."

I remember Mme. Nutron, wife of a doctor of science, in whose home I lived while on a visit to France. When she cleaned her three-story house from 8:00 to 11:00 each morning, she was always singing. She understood that the act of changing something that is dirty into something that is clean is real joy; it is creation itself. Pleasure-seeking, by contrast, is not joy for there is no true creativity in it. Joy is the result of change, and women are in a position to bask in this kind of joy.

Chapter 4

Expanding the Family

Sex

I have not discussed sexual life for good reason. If you follow the Order of Nature, your sexual life will become orderly. If it is *out* of order, we can conclude that your whole life is the same, and especially in the realm of eating.

The consequences of disorder in diet and general living are many and varied. One sad result is the need for birth control on the part of men or women by internal or external means. Another is the overly masculine young lady who has an excess of hair on various parts of her body or the feminized young boy who has no hair at all. Such people are certain to be unhappy.

If a husband and wife are healthy and have a proper balance of yin (expansive) and yang (contractive) factors in their diet and surroundings, they will give birth to equal numbers of boys and girls. If all the children are girls, the family is too extravagant and eating too richly. Such a family will see tragedy or unhappiness. It is a better indication if all of the offspring are boys. Alternation, however, is best — boy, girl, boy, girl, etc.

The apparently healthy woman who cannot conceive is not balancing her food well. Her diet is usually very high in fruit or sugar and other confections. Yet she need not give up hope even if she has not conceived for ten years. If she starts eating macrobiotically, she will soon be able to have a baby.

Many women today submit to abortion in spite of the fact that it can spoil their health. Poor health and sadness are the guilty burden of those who go against the law of nature. This is true Justice.

Heredity

At this point I should like to discuss the modern theory of heredity and criticize it from the standpoint of macrobiotics.

Modern baby care is based on the theory of heredity, a hypothesis and as-yet unproven concept. Darwin's theory of evolution is similar in that we cannot accept it as a positive truth – it is also in the hypothetical stage. Just as Malthus's theory of population has disappeared, so will both the heredity and evolution theories fade into disuse because they are not based on a concrete, fundamental principle. How can we discuss life or health on the basis of such flimsy suppositions?

The heredity theory, for example, proposes that we marry a genetically sound individual in order to produce a healthy baby. In theory, a person's faulty genes demand that he choose a mate who is as unfortunate as he is; he may even decide not to marry at all if he takes this concept seriously enough. Thinking of this sort is too egoistic and produces tragic results — for example, a mother killing the baby that she feels is basically unsound.

The same theory suggests that character is inherited, that weak parents make a weak child. But even healthy parents can produce a weak child, while weak parents have produced many a healthy one. If weak character is inherited, if such is the legacy of an infant, God must be unfair because such an infant has trouble all his life without deserving it. He is punished without having ever committed a crime.

I believe that God is absolutely fair in every sense of the word. God gives us life, and health is the true condition for that life. God gives everyone health. Just look at nature! All creatures seem capable of adapting to their environment and remaining healthy; they never create unnatural things or deformity. Only human beings, the *conquerors* of nature, lose their health and produce these things or situations that are unnatural.

There is no proof whatever for the dogmatic assertion that certain illnesses are inherited. Myopia (near-sightedness) is a case in point. It would seem that the whole idea of heredity serves as nothing more than an elaborate camouflage for a fundamental ignorance of the cause of illness. I cannot agree with the theory, simply because I have seen so many of the diseases labeled as hereditary respond to natural food.

It is said that an individual's constitution is inherited, be it weak or healthy. Yet a healthy person can produce a weak child. Why? Modern medicine, without having given the subject the deep thought it merits, has grasped at the opportunity to avoid the whole problem by calling early weakness in the human being congenital. But after all, what is "congenital"? Is it hereditary? What is "hereditary"? Is it congenital? I patiently await the time when someone will explain the mechanism of heredity. I have not yet met the man who could.

The genetic theory suggests that a child's character is inherited from its parents. If this were true, every scholar's child would be wise, a beauty's child would be lovely to look at, and the son of a nearsighted man would have bad eyes. Our lives, predetermined, would always be as miserable as those of our parents. We can, however, be happy in the thought that a scholar can produce a dullard, a criminal can sire a saint, and a blind man can father an infant with perfect eyes.

In most cases, a baby has no knowledge of delinquency, is immune to sickness, and is never nearsighted. On the contrary, he is farsighted and can see the stars and sun very clearly. With growth, however, his line of sight shortens and he progressively sees best those things that are closest to him.

All people start from the same point. It is only through *diet* and much *effort* that they become scholars, saints, or big businessmen.

Modern medicine is alarmed by birth defects but the macrobiotic person is not; he knows that diet can correct them. Furthermore, he knows that the child of a macrobiotic woman will not have them. For example, if a baby has sores that run continuously, modern medicine suggests treatment that alleviates the symptom but never actually cures the patient. The macrobiotic diet, however, heals diseases at their source.

Experience over thousands of years indicates that all congenital weakness is caused by the mother since it is the food that she takes in that determines how her baby will develop. This is true for syphilis as well as any other disease the baby may have at birth.

My sole reason for mentioning heredity at all is to do what I can to quiet the fears of those women who are so anxious because of prevalent scientific theories.

Pregnancy

Life becomes more complicated as the factory of happiness expands. It gives birth to its first product — a lovely baby. The creation of new life is so difficult that to take care of that life is our most important job. Should we fail at this task we can know no happiness at all.

Preparation for the production of a strong and happy baby begins *before* pregnancy. About forty years ago, the mortality rate for infants in Japan was 255,000 per year — one death every two minutes. The generally accepted cause for this tragedy was birth defects. Yet the fact that these birth defects went hand in hand with the careless diet and disordered life of the mothers, both before and during pregnancy, was completely overlooked.

Death Rate from Birth Defects in Osaka, Japan

(Note that the increase in birth defects parallels the popularity or acceptance of Western nutrition in Japan.)

Year	Number of Deaths
1925	1598
1926	1604
1927	1547
1928	2283
1929	2085
1930	2107
1931	2200
1932	2230
1933	2622
1934	2663
1935	3117

Macrobiotics is not merely another point of view regarding nutrition, or just another opinion in a field overrun with theories about calories, vitamins, minerals, and economics. Its essence is humble gratitude and appreciation for that which produces food — sun, earth, air, water, energy, the metabolism of the universe, and the effort expended by all of humanity or society.

To feel this gratitude and have such an understanding of nature and the source of life during pregnancy has always been considered of fundamental importance in the Orient. It was called *taikyo* or "education for pregnancy" by the early Chinese saints, and was known by the same name in Japan. This education has been forgotten in the modern world because people have grown to be more concerned with pleasure, taste, or calories. Their outlook on life is predominantly materialistic; they have forgotten about gratitude and spirituality. This is why the modern generation rarely produces offspring whose mental and physical conditions are well-balanced.

One of the basic precepts of *taikyo* deals with the atmosphere that surrounds a pregnant woman. The understanding is that she should read a book of religious or moral teaching each morning. She should not look at strong colors or come into contact with other strong stimuli. She should not look at cruel things or read stories about cruelty.

It is interesting that even in France it is said that pregnant women had better not go to the cinema or drama or read novels of any kind. In modern times, unfortunately, both the Orient and the Occident have forgotten this ancient wisdom. If you deeply desire to have a happy, healthy baby, you would be well-advised to follow this teaching.

* * *

During pregnancy, a woman's diet must be more strict than ever because the destiny of her child is being determined. In nine months, the primary cell multiplies three billion times. (By way of contrast, our weight multiplies only twenty times from birth to the age of twenty.) All the evolutionary biological transformations are re-enacted during that period: monocell, plankton, algae, fish, slug, leech, invertebrate, reptile, monkey, etc. During this time, the fetus is fed only by what its mother eats. If that food has been correct, a strong baby will be born.

Since the eyes, ears, nose, mouth, and all other physical characteristics are being formed at this time, they are directly affected by the mother's diet. If the mother eats fish every day, the baby's nose will be flat. If she eats more vegetables than grains, or if she eats meat very often, the ear is small and without a lobe. This is called a "poor man's ear" in Japan. The person with such an ear can become very unhappy and at times very destructive. A good ear is large, has a lobe, and is flat against the head. The baby with an ear like this can become a great man.

The woman who produces a child with a triangular nose which has a base equal to the width of the mouth; deep, quiet eyes; and large ears; has good reason for being happy.

If a woman bears twins, triplets, or quadruplets; if her baby is born feet first; if a woman cannot conceive; she can only blame herself and her poor diet.

If you follow the macrobiotic principle and encounter any one of these problems, you can easily correct it. Best of all, it is not likely that they will ever arise in the first place because you will have made yourself immune to them through macrobiotics. This even applies to those diseases that a parent carries. They will *not* be transmitted to the child. Modern medicine cannot explain what is referred to as "immunity." Macrobiotically speaking, it is produced by righteous food. He who eats righteous food never worries about syphilis or gonorrhea. Babies are free from all such diseases if the mother has eaten correctly. Fortunately, those infants who do suffer from them can be healed completely by macrobiotic food.

Diet During Pregnancy.   The main food should be brown rice, organically grown in your immediate area if possible. If there is no brown rice available, use rye, millet, buckwheat, corn, or any whole grain cereal which has been eaten traditionally in that area.

The side dishes should consist of vegetables in season, sauteed. Eat four to five mouthfuls of cereal for each mouthful of vegetables. It is best to avoid potatoes, tomatoes, and eggplant.

Never use fruit (raw or cooked), sugar, candy, ice cream, or dairy products.

Have miso soup once each day.

Never use meat.

You may eat fish occasionally. When you do, choose small fish and eat them whole. Discard no parts and always cook three times more vegetables than fish. When cooking either fish or vegetables, do not discard any part. Use the skin and bones of the fish, the root of the vegetable.

Use *koi-koku* (carp soup) or salted salmon cooked with hiziki, kombu (two varieties of seaweed), and a very small amount of bamboo shoot (available in the United States in canned form only); plus the dish called *kinpira*. A combination of aduki beans and kombu seaweed would also be very good.

Pickled foods are acceptable provided that they have been in brine (salt only, no vinegar!) for a very long time, e.g., daikon radishes that have been pickled for three years, umeboshi plums that have been in salt for three years, or raw vegetables that have been pickled in *miso* (soy bean paste) for two to three years.

Eat new pickles only during the hot summer; even then take only one or two ounces per meal. Some people recommend fresh pickles or fruit salad as a source of vitamin C. I am very sad to hear this because they can be a source of great danger to both mother and fetus.

Do not eat desserts that are very yin (expansive), i.e., those containing sugar, honey, or artificial sweeteners. If you like desserts, eat the following:

a. brown rice *mochi* (pounded rice cake) dusted with soy-bean flour;
b. brown rice mochi baked with tamari soy sauce;
c. brown rice mochi combined with mugwort (a wild grass);
d. sweet rice cooked with aduki beans;
e. *sushi* (rice rolled in nori seaweed) without vinegar;
f. thick aduki soup with added salt, mochi and winter squash.

Do not eat between meals with the possible exception of items listed directly above.

Do not drink more than sixteen ounces of liquid per day. Brown rice tea, brown rice soup, grain coffee, and grain milk (*kokkoh*) are very good.[2]

The following foods should not be taken: tuna, sardines, shrimp, crab, and mackerel (cooked, canned, or fresh) since they are too yang (contractive); all fruits, sugar, cakes, tomatoes, potatoes, eggplant, and ice because they are too yin (expansive).

When eating, posture should be good — sit erect. Before beginning a meal give thanks for *everything* including your food.

Chew all foods very well, especially brown rice — *100 times* per mouthful.

Staying Well During Pregnancy.   Physical activity every day is a necessity — any sort of housework will do.

An occasional hip bath with the dried leaves of daikon radish can be very helpful. Cook two or three bunches of dried leaves plus a handful of salt in one gallon of water. Sit in a tub filled with enough hot water to cover the body to the waist. Add strained cooked mixture at intervals so the bath will remain strong and hot.

If you follow the macrobiotic diet, you will suffer from neither morning sickness nor swollen legs. The individual who has not eaten carefully and who has developed swollen legs can use a ginger compress on them two or three times a day. Kinpira, kombu, and aduki beans are specifics for such a condition.

If morning sickness does occur, the treatment depends upon the woman's constitution. Women with yin constitutions (very white skin, low body temperature, slow pulse, those who cannot stand hot baths, and whose movements and speech are slow) should prepare a special drink in the following manner:

Scrape the burnt-on carbon from an earthenware frying pan. Put one teaspoonful of the scrapings in one cup of boiled water and allow to settle for ten minutes. Drink the top liquid only — do *not* drink the sediment. This is a Chinese medicine called *fukuryukan*.[3]

Yang women (red skin color, short temper, quick pulse, those who have a liking for hot baths) had better drink three or four ounces of fresh orange juice once or twice a day until their condition changes.

Delivery

Since delivery is a natural physiological phenomenon, it should not be painful. If you carefully follow the macrobiotic way, you can have a beautiful baby quickly and easily. It is even likely that your child will be born long before the midwife has arrived on the scene!

The woman who does have a painfully difficult delivery has been eating incorrectly; the child born of such a delivery may very likely be an unhappy one.

We have all heard of farm women both in Japan and in other parts of the world who easily give birth while working in the fields. This is difficult to comprehend if one is unaware of the importance of good diet.

The best positions for delivery are sitting and squatting. They permit the baby to emerge naturally in its own way. You can stay in bed two to five days after delivery. It is best to tighten the belt[4] after delivery and sleep with a low pillow under the head.

Women should wear light clothes before, during and after delivery.

After delivery, the mother should eat strengthening foods such as miso soup with mochi; rice kayu with umeboshi (salted plum) or miso; and rice balls with sesame salt. Three or four days after delivery she should take *tekka*. Vegetables should include scallions and daikon radish. In the morning she should eat miso soup with mochi.[5]

Experience in Japan has shown that the above kind of food produces the rapid healing and return to normal of the ovaries.

Chapter 5

Baby Care

There is no special knowledge or study required as preparation for taking care of a baby. Even animals care for their young without a doctor or any special training, yet their offspring are strong and rarely die while young. Modern medicine teaches that we should take special precautions such as keeping the room warm and providing warm clothing. This is a very big mistake that weakens the child. A baby should wear light clothing and go outdoors for one or two hours each day even during the winter. Its room should *not* be especially warm.

The care given a child by its mother is the first step in its education, the foundation of its character.

Even though a new baby is fragile and difficult to handle, *only* its mother should bathe it — not a nurse, midwife, or relative. This activity will give the mother a great and unforgettable pleasure.

The most important thing to remember is not to pamper the child. Even if it is crying, a child should not be held other than to give it milk.

While nursing, the mother must study, read, or think. Above all, she should not allow herself to be controlled by her child. When it has been fed, the baby should be left alone. A child that cries when it is not hungry must be ill; again we find the fault in its mother's incorrect diet.

Never allow bed-wetting and dispense with diapers after the child is three days old. You will learn to recognize the signs of its need to eliminate — they usually occur after waking, and if you become aware of them you will encounter no difficulties.

Give your child as few toys as possible. Never give inflammable toys.

The best type of clothing for a child is cotton because it strengthens the skin. If the cloth is dyed, the dye should be natural and never of the harmful type. White cotton cloth that is light and loose is best.

Children should never be bound tight like a package. They are yang (active and aggressive) and must have the freedom to move.

A macrobiotic child is free from toothaches, diphtheria, pneumonia, and the other usual children's diseases. He is usually easy to raise — a joyful, happy jewel in the family. His young mother is happy because by raising such a child she is contributing in a large way to the process of building a happy life.

Appearance of the Infant

A healthy baby should be red and small. If its skin color is white or green, it will have an unhappy and troubled life. If you are not macrobiotic, there is a good chance that you will have such a baby. Nevertheless, you have no need to worry. An understanding of macrobiotics will enable you to change your infant's color to a healthy red.

Recently, a large French newspaper analyzed a phenomenon that no one can explain: the human race is growing progressively taller. The average length and weight of babies at birth is also increasing. Why is this? Anyone who has studied the Unique Principle has the means of solving this problem. Large babies are more yin, reflecting an increase in yin foods in the diet of the mothers.

Up to the age of six years, the macrobiotic child is smaller than others. He takes long in learning to walk, his body is thin and muscular, and he is quick, calm and alert. From the age of six, he begins growing at a normal rate.

A large body is not necessarily a sign of health. Remember: spiritual growth can be infinite. Physiological growth has its natural limits. The larger the body, the smaller the spirit.

An infant's hair should be fair and soft at birth. If during pregnancy, however, the mother has taken much fruit, tomato/cucumber salads, or other yin foods, the hair will be hard and dark. The body must be small, red, and hard. If there is a birthmark it should be on the buttock. Fingernails should be long. The infant should weigh between four and one-half and five pounds and must cry strongly — the louder the better. It is not good, however, for a baby to cry unnecessarily as it will when left alone. Hunger should be its only reason for crying.

Feeding the Newborn

There is no need to feed an infant during the first twenty or thirty hours after birth, so do not be alarmed if it cries during this time. Under most circumstances the crying is only an expression of the need to eliminate.

The breast-feeding macrobiotic mother does not need to sterilize her nipples, and usually produces just enough milk for her child. If for some reason she does not have enough, cow's milk is not advisable as a substitute. It is impossible to grow a strong child on the milk of another animal. The milk of a cow is designed specifically for her calves.

The woman with insufficient milk should eat macrobiotically, taking *koi-koku* (carp soup),[6] as well as miso soup with mochi. Western medicine, in this case, recommends fruit and much vegetable and animal protein in order to increase the quantity of milk and raise the vitamin level. Please do not be deceived by this erroneous idea. Excess fruits or vegetables may produce more milk but it will be thin, watery, and not very nutritious.

* * *

The popular belief is that nursing will ruin a woman's figure; the macrobiotic viewpoint is that a woman who ages as a result of nursing is not eating correctly. A macrobiotic mother becomes progressively more feminine. Figures notwithstanding, what is of prime importance is the fact that even a sick mother's milk is better for her baby than cow's milk. Only a cold-hearted woman could resist nursing in the face of this knowledge.

If the mother is unable to nurse, the best substitute for her milk is special rice cream or *kokkoh*.[7] An infant can have as much of these foods as it desires.

Weaning and Solid Foods

Nursing is to be stopped after one year or when the child begins to teethe since the emergence of teeth indicates that the time has come for baby to begin chewing. Those mothers who allow a child to nurse after this time will weaken its character and cause it to become egoistic and exclusive.

When breast-feeding is stopped, grain milk without salt will be the best substitute. Grain milk, cooked in a covered pan for at least one hour on low heat and an asbestos pad, will be easily assimilated by the child.

After the fifth month, one of the daily meals should be a cereal cream made of rice, barley, wheat, oats or millet, cooked three to four hours without salt, in four volumes of water. If salt is needed, it is better to add two or three drops of tamari soy sauce or a pinch of gomasio to the bowl after the grain is cooked. To the cereal cream, add ten percent of vegetables steamed in their own juice in a covered pan, and very lightly salted. Onion, carrots, leeks, pumpkins, and cabbage may be used. Finish with a tablespoon of carrot juice or a small amount (one teaspoon) of raw apple, a tablespoon of apple-sauce or a small piece of baked apple.

If the infant does not gain weight due to poor digestion, the mother will have to chew and salivate thoroughly each meal before giving it to the baby.

At seven months, the baby will be taught mastication by chewing on whole grain bread crust or a rice cake. (Incidentally, it is very bad to give a six- or seven-month-old infant crackers or biscuits containing sugar or any sweetening.) During teething, a rice ball or a piece of daikon pickle to chew on is very helpful.

In the evening, the baby will enjoy strained vegetable soup thickened with some barley cream, wheat cream, rice or oat cream, some whole wheat spaghetti or a well-cooked whole wheat bread soup. Break whole grain bread in pieces and cover with boiling water, cook for forty-five minutes, and add a small amount of strained or pureed vegetables, or a small amount of grated apple.

A small amount of raw vegetables is a valuable source of yin which will give the child strength and will help his growth. At the beginning, give a tablespoon of carrot juice with a pinch of gomasio or a drop of tamari soy sauce. Later, when the baby has teeth, substitute raw grated carrot for the juice, two or three small radishes, three or four slices of cucumber, chopped lettuce, parsley, or dandelion when in season.

At a later age, children may be served dandelion, spinach, watercress, turnips, oysterplants, string beans, or fresh soybeans, cut small and cooked for a short time (*nitsuke* style). Some recipe variations make for easier menus.

Oven-baked vegetables are suitable for the whole family. It is only necessary to yangize them more for the adults by adding, at the end of cooking time, a small amount of tamari soy sauce or diluted miso.

Place pumpkin cut in one-quarter-inch cubes, whole carrots, and whole onions in a Pyrex dish. Sprinkle a small amount of sea salt on the vegetables. If the vegetables are too dry, moisten at the start with a tablespoon of water. Bake in medium oven (350 degrees) for forty-five minutes to one hour. For a child, puree the cooked vegetables with a fork. For the adult, cut into small slivers or slices.

Side dishes for youngsters consist of vegetables — never fish, meat, eggs, milk or other animal products.

However, there are times when the baby will refuse all vegetable dishes and only accept cereals. The mother should not worry or try to force some vegetables. This will prove useless since the child is not at all interested.

As the child grows, his food horizon may be broadened. From the time his teeth appear, he will chew drier rice (cooked with less water), waffles, pancakes and cakes made at home with whole grain flours, and wheat or rye breads. Liquids should be offered only after the meal: rice tea, three-year tea, spring water. Mu tea should not be given to children.

When the child is one year old, the proportion of vegetables in the main meal may be increased to twenty or thirty percent. A dessert may be made of cereal cream to which is added a few raisins or currants or one-fourth of a chopped apple.

Order of Eating

To begin a meal by drinking fruit juices is very detrimental. Even though it is now in fashion, it kills the natural appetite.

Soup may be taken at the beginning of a meal as it is always slightly salty.

A meal must begin with yang food and end with yin food. X-rays have shown that if a meal is started with yin — salad, fruit, coffee, cakes, juices, etc. — all of these foods remain undigested. Often these will be forcefully eliminated by diarrhea or vomiting. If only a lump of sugar is eaten before a meal, the whole meal goes undigested; as it passes into the intestine, it creates gases and bad odors.

Salt

The most important of all considerations in the feeding of a child is the amount of salt given. Caution should be exercised to make certain that it is no more than *one-tenth* of an adult's daily requirements.

Too much or too little salt retards the development of the child. But how does one determine the right amount? Bowel movements are important. They should be yellow-orange in color. If they are too light, white or green, a salt deficiency is indicated. If they are dark or hard, there is an excess of salt. The feces should come away from the diaper by simple soaking and should never be sticky.

If you coat the end of your finger with finely crushed sea salt and the baby sucks that finger with relish, he needs salt. You have not been salting his bottle enough. On the other hand, if a child craves too much water or too much yin food, it only means that his food is too salty. At this point, instead of refusing the yin or the water, you only need to reduce the child's intake of salt.

Remember, a few grains of salt can change everything.

Illness in Children

A child's condition is reflected in the condition of its stool. Elimination should be punctual and of a good consistency —never soft or green. Diapers should be easy to clean without soap. If a nursing child has diarrhea or bad-smelling green evacuations, its mother's diet must be checked immediately.

If the top of a baby's head, the fontanel, has not closed after a year and a half has passed, its mother's milk has been imperfect. I know of one boy whose fontanel had not closed after nine years with the result that he could not attend school. After six months of macrobiotic eating, he recovered completely.

It is very seldom necessary to give specific "remedies" to children. At all times, it is better to remember which food was consumed on the preceding day. If there was an excess of yin given — desserts, fruit or drinks — it is only necessary to eliminate these and everything will return to normal. In extreme cases, a kuzu preparation can be given.

Excess yang can also cause a cold. In that case, give rice without salt, cream of rice, or, in extreme cases, a small amount of cooked apple.

Diarrhea. Feed the child polished white rice for a day. Be sure to wash raw rice to remove sugar or glucose coating. If diarrhea continues, dissolve a tablespoon of kuzu in a bowl of cold water, add one small umeboshi plum or half a large one, two tablespoons of tamari soy sauce and cook gently until liquid is clear. Give one-fourth of the bowl for infants and one-half bowl for an older child.

Constipation. Give well-cooked aduki beans, pureed.

Worms. Once a month, give strong mugwort tea. Boil a four-inch twig for one-half hour in one cup of water. Boil until liquid is half evaporated. The child should drink this tea upon arising in the morning.

Earaches. Mix one part sesame oil and one part ginger (powder or juice). Heat the mixture until lukewarm and use a spoon to drip into the ear. Relief is instantaneous.

Fever. Give the child a bath with water at the exact temperature of the child, e.g., body temperature of 101 degrees, bathwater at 101 degrees.

Bruises, Wounds and Scratches. Apply boiled salted water. Outdoors, for small scratches, clean with saliva.

*   *   *

In healing a sick child, the mother must rely on the infant's instinct, on the nature of its bowel movements and on her own good sense. Above all, it is her judgment that counts. Good intentions, sentiment, and the mechanical application of macrobiotic knowledge are not enough. One must think, know what life is and understand the Unique Principle.

The Joy of Parenthood

How joyful it is to witness the growth of new life, be it that of a child, a plant, or an animal. The growth of a human being is most amusing, however, since this tiny being plays with you, understands you, studies you, and gives you courage and strength when you are troubled.

You can enjoy a truly happy life only if you have a child. This is so obvious if one spends some time at a sanitarium like one that I visited in Europe, an old-age home for childless, lonely people. It is very depressing.

How sad it is to give up having children only because you do not want to take the trouble to raise them. The individual who avoids parenthood because he wants the freedom to enjoy himself or because his income is low is a coward. True, child care is a large responsibility and very often a lot of trouble, but if you avoid such responsibility or difficulty, you will never understand or enjoy pleasure, gratitude, or happiness.

Happiness only comes to those who tolerate unhappiness.

Chapter 6

Childhood

From the very beginning the mother should not yield to the whims of the baby. He should be allowed to play by himself, left to cry if he does not succeed in his attempts, etc. When the child begins to talk, to understand, his games and everyday experiences must be utilized to teach him the Unique Principle of yin and yang. Later on, this teaching will be continued from the questions he will ask on his own.

Co-education

In schools, it is imperative that boys and girls be kept separate. When boys and girls are taught together, sexuality is destroyed.

Sex is yin and yang. This yin and yang must stay separate in order that one day they may be attracted to each other and combine very strongly.

If hunger is physical appetite, then sex drive is biological appetite. We know that appetite is caused by absence of food, thirst by lack of drink. It is necessary to be without love in order to love.

Also of importance is that the young male child should not touch his mother's clothing. The young boy should always be seated next to his father. This not only strengthens his masculine sexuality but also helps the child break the bond with his mother and begin his relationship with the world at large.

Diet for the Older Child

If the mother has eaten properly during pregnancy, and if

the child has had a balanced diet from birth to the age of six, he will instinctively know which foods agree with him and will seldom take more food than necessary. If one offers sugar to a child who has been nourished macrobiotically during the embryological period, he will spit it out. He instinctively understands the harmful effects sugar has on his organism. If one offers him fruit, he will choose those that are most yang: apples, strawberries, and cherries. He shows faultless judgment.

Children should not be given animal products until they have reached the age of fifteen or sixteen years. In fact, it is better not to give any animal food at all to insure the highest development of thinking power.

Modern nutrition recommends fruit and dairy products without reservation. This is questionable since these foods in quantity are too yin (expansive) for the average human organism. But there is still another consideration — the social one. All the land area of our globe is not sufficient to produce enough of these things to feed the population of the earth. Sooner or later we will have to face the consequences of the bad judgment that gave birth to this idea.

Cattle grazing and the growing of fruit are far less economical than grain and vegetable cultivation. From the social standpoint, the theory is unfair — it is without social justice.

There are no animals in nature other than man that take milk after they have begun to teethe. They seem to understand instinctively that milk is only for an infant with no teeth. The child who continues to take milk until it is four or five years old will have a mineral deficiency — weak bones.[8] Excessive use of cow's milk renders the human child prone to meningitis in adolescence.

Modern nutrition theories advise that our diet should provide an abundance of vitamin C, vitamin D, and calcium, but our ancestors (especially the scholars and monks) never took such things and enjoyed wonderful health.

I do not deny the importance of vitamins or calcium; I am not against the theories of modern nutrition in the least. I merely say that such a concept of nutrition, physiology, or life is incomplete and that we cannot rely upon it as the basis for establishing health. Surely no important scholar in modern physiology or nutrition can say that modern nutrition is perfect; most of them, in fact, have observed that it is quite the opposite. Within ten years, therefore, present theories are sure to change dramatically if what has occurred in the past ten years is any indication.

Modern nutritionists do not even agree on the amount of vitamins necessary for health, despite the fact that it is common knowledge that such things can be dangerous if taken in too large or small a quantity. Oxygen, for instance, is very important to life, but if it is taken in insufficient or excessive amounts it can be fatal. Magnesium, too, is important, but an excess of one-half gram is lethal.

Modern science does not yet fully understand nutrition or physiology. It does not know what life is; science is therefore incomplete. For us to rely on such incomplete theories as a guide to health and full life can be extremely dangerous.

Even if the correct amount of vitamins, magnesium, or calcium necessary to sustain life were ever to be decided upon, we still could not live on these alone. Life is larger than just the analytical understanding of its parts. For example, the airplane is an important strategic weapon, yet an army cannot rely upon it alone. It is but one part of a fighting force that consists of many components — men, ships, tanks, guns, supply sources, etc.

It is very simple to care for a child if we follow macrobiotic eating and drinking habits. Sugar, bananas, tomatoes, potatoes, etc., are not traditional food in the Northern Hemisphere; they are of tropical origin.

Exercise and Play

There exists a modern superstition to the effect that tall, fat people are healthy and that short, thin people are weak and sick. I call this a superstition because vigorous athletes with magnificent physiques and enlarged muscles seem to die early while the short, thin weaklings often go on and on. Size apparently is not one of the main criteria of health.

Gymnastics and exercises are unnecessary for children because family life can provide sufficient activity to make them strong. They can be given chores such as sweeping, mopping, or helping mother in whatever way is possible. In this way, a child learns tolerance as well as how to care for and respect his environment.

In France, I had a writer friend named Kukyu whose wife was a school principal. Of their two children, the daughter always played alone. She had few toys but was happy. Her greatest joy was a piece of cloth that she changed into an endless number of playthings through the use of her imagination. She played with this cloth so much that she was called "Chiffon."

Training such as this is good for children because it develops harmony and unity within the home. I feel that it is most necessary because it is so practical. In rich families where there are servants, where the children have too many toys and no practical training like chores, inventive playing, or hardship, they develop into melancholy, nervous, sentimental, unhappy, weak adults. Such tragedies are the direct product of a mother's sentimentality in raising her children.

* * *

Scholars have written at length about child care and diet but their methods are usually very involved and difficult to put into practice. What we suggest in macrobiotics, by contrast, is plain and simple. Many people wonder, "Can this be true? Is it so easy?" All I can offer as an answer is this: look at animals in their natural surroundings — they live simply and eat plain, unadulterated food. Consider the men who come from poor background and have little care as children — they manage to become strong, important people. Individuals from rich backgrounds who have had many things given to them, including fancy food, tend to become weak and spoiled.

Birds never plant or harvest. They are always busy, joyfully flying about and singing, yet they are always fed. In autumn they eat dry grass; in winter they find food in the snow. They are healthy even in the coldest weather, never troubled by heart disease, tuberculosis or colds.

There is an old saying in China: "The best wood does not grow in rich soil." Strong wood thrives in the mountains where the soil is poor and it is windy and cold. Wood easily grown in rich soil is weak because it is not subjected to the changes in weather that foster strength and endurance. Human life is the same. If you want your child to be a strong man who can bear the burdens of life in this world, give him natural food and simple surroundings. Lincoln, Franklin and many other great men were raised in this manner.

This is the secret of child care. You will be well rewarded if you use it.

How wonderful it is if we are poor. In the words of the Bible, "The rich cannot enter the Kingdom of Heaven." Give up the desire for wealth, comfort, and pleasure, for true happiness comes only to the humble, simple, just people in this life.

We are children of nature. In macrobiotics the belief is that to follow the Order of the Universe is happiness itself. The unhappy, the sick, and the ignorant are criminals who have disregarded and violated that Order.

I believe in the orderliness of nature. To follow it is to pay the premium on one's life insurance. One can become the eternal child.

Chapter 7

The Age of Activity

During our early years, our comprehension and judgment are weak and unclear because of sentimentality. When we begin to be active in society, near the age of twenty, we must study the principle of Life that can establish our judgment securely on *all* levels, since it is vital that we be able to think clearly about food, profession, and life itself.

If we have been raised macrobiotically, there is no need for special instruction — our development will be in the right direction, and our judgment will be good enough to handle any circumstances that may arise.

Today's public education, unfortunately, is far removed from this kind of teaching. The job falls to the parents, as it always has, to provide the child with a conception of nature and of the universe; to point the way to an understanding of the relationship of nature and the universe to Life — the relationship of the parts to the whole. If a child has been taught these basic fundamentals, he can be depended upon to judge capably for himself in his everyday living.

The kind of education that I advocate has two phases:

a. providing the right food and drink, and
b. teaching the principle by which health and happiness can be established and maintained.

Any other knowledge must be acquired by the individual through specific study on his own.

In view of this, it would be interesting and valuable for high school history classes to investigate the relationship between food and the rise and fall of nations.

Since modern education deals largely with the assimilation and memorization of facts, the individual loses his ability to think and act independently. It is thus not a *true* education.

Young people of twenty must develop a confident attitude that says, "I will never be sick." With it they can lead strong lives, take any job, and happily meet any difficulty whatsoever.

If they are brought up in a macrobiotic household on a balanced diet but do not have an understanding of the fundamental principle involved — the relationship of food to life — they will encounter great difficulties. This is particularly true if it becomes necessary for them to change their environment or function in a different culture. The Japanese are an example of this. Traditionally, they ate a good macrobiotic diet but, along the way, they lost or forgot the guiding principle from which that diet developed. The result was that with the introduction of Western medicine into Japan, they abandoned their tradition and lost their health at the same time.

If a person is raised macrobiotically until the age of twenty, he can eat anything after that, because his judgment will enable him to choose his food carefully, easily, and without worry.

A man's diet must change according to his profession. In Japan, for example, people eat grains and vegetables primarily. Those who do physical labor, however, take some animal food, principally fish — about ten percent of the total food intake. This is not an absolute essential, however, even for laborers. Rather than being an actual necessity, it is more a pleasure item to satisfy the taste.

Those who do mental or intellectual work should eat only grains and vegetables — *no animal food*. This includes office workers, writers, scholars, students, executives, men of religion or leaders in any field.

Do not make the mistake of considering macrobiotics to be merely another variety of puritanism or dogma; it is neither pro-vegetarianism nor anti-carnivorism. *We do not deny one kind of food or praise another.* We teach the relationship between man and the Universe, and offer the principle that is essential if we are to understand and become one with the

Infinite, God or nature. Macrobiotics might more correctly be called a new interpretation of naturalism.

The person who is macrobiotic appears to be highly selective in his choice of food. In his own eyes, however, he eats *anything* that he desires of God's food and really desires *none* of the man-made variety.

Just consider fruit trees — they are no longer God's product. They are forced by men to produce long after they might either have died naturally or have been destroyed by insects. They are kept alive past their prime by artificial methods that render them unfit as food for human beings.

Macrobiotics offers a practical way of establishing health in one's life. Its fundamental idea is that as long as nature exists, health is possible. Since food is given by nature (God), if we eat in accord with nature, we are inevitably healthy and happy. Nature gives many things but *we must choose what is good for us.* The art of making such a choice is macrobiotics.

Some people will wonder how such a simple principle can ensure health, cure sickness, and help us to enjoy life. Such people must look at nature; it is all around them. Any animal, bird, insect, flower, tree or plant is full of health and happiness, eating only what God has made.

Animal foods, fruit, and sugar are not essential to life and should be used only for pleasure or medication. They are all enemies of activity, with sugar being by far the most destructive.

It is easy to become addicted to these foods, so if you crave them, be careful. Those who always want coffee or alcohol are not as far removed from the plight of the drug addict as they might like to believe. Strict macrobiotics have no need for such taste stimulation; they do not want such foods and are not addicted to them. Those who are not free from such cravings and sensations are not happy; they are sick. If you are not free, you cannot be healthy. A healthy person accepts the most simple food as having the best taste. This kind of acceptance is the aim of macrobiotics. With this flexibility, you can be most active in your adult life.

Chapter 8

Old Age

We have all heard people say, "I am getting old." As a child I thought, "What a strange thing to say!" The same phrase later on in my life made me think, "How poor man is!"

At the age of forty, I was startled to feel weakness in my body. "I am beginning to get old," I thought, since in Japan it is said that old age begins when pain and stiffness appear, somewhere between the ages of forty and forty-five.

My feeling of age was not the result of macrobiotics but of the circumstances of my early life. As a youth, I had lived and eaten poorly, studying all the time. Later I worked as a sailor on the Indian Ocean. My Arabian crewmates, raised in a tropical country and possessing very strong constitutions, thrived on the hard work we did. I had grown up in a much different climate so the combination of ocean, labor, and diet not only made me very sickly but caused what I felt to be "old age."

After a very long voyage, I returned to Japan and recovered my strength by eating delicious brown rice. From that time on I have never felt tired, nor have I ever had the need to rest. In fact, as long as I am awake I am at work. I easily fulfill three conditions for good health:

1. no fatigue
2. good appetite
3. good sleep.

How could I feel anything but gratitude for my twenty years of macrobiotics?

The first ten years were full of mistakes. Sometimes I took

too much salt; at other times, not enough. I experienced much failure. Though the last five years of my long stay in Paris were spent under the poorest of living conditions, I have now re-established good health. Whereas long ago I could not smoke or drink, I can now do either as I like. I enjoy any cuisine — Western, Chinese, Japanese, or Indian. I like fruit, candy, chocolate, and whiskey very much. If I choose to use these things now, I am able to avoid harm because I can balance yin and yang.

I have told you this because many people think that macrobiotics is a twentieth century variety of stoicism. *But he who cannot drink, smoke, eat fruit or meat is a cripple.* Macrobiotics is a way to build health that enables us to eat and drink anything we like, whenever we like, without being obsessed or driven to do so. Macrobiotics is not a negative way of living. It is positive, creative, artistic, religious, and philosophical.

I never get sick now. I do not wear an overcoat in cold or wet weather and I sleep with an open window the whole year round. My only trouble is that I do too much work, yet it is very hard for me to stop because I take much salt every day.

Since I am only fifty years old, I am not sure that I am qualified to speak on the subject of old age. Because of my years of experience in the realm of macrobiotics, however, I will at least try.

Macrobiotically speaking, old age begins at seventy. At this time an individual should

1. reduce his salt intake;
2. make certain that his food is as simple as possible;
3. take vegetable oils daily in small amounts.

There is no special diet in old age for the person who has had a macrobiotic childhood and youth. He can eat anything because many years of macrobiotic living have left him well balanced physiologically, psychologically, and economically. He is not pushed or driven; he is relaxed and fulfilled.

The macrobiotics of old age amounts to simply this: *live in nature.* Enjoy cold in winter, accept heat in summer, admire flowers in spring, and write poems in autumn. Live in nature with a calm, quiet spirit. Give to others of your happiness, for old age is the most happy time of life.

I recall a very fitting poem by the German poet Lautenbach. It describes an oak tree that has withstood several hundred years of buffeting by all kinds of weather — wind, rain, storm, frost, and snow. It is a very tall tree with wide, strong branches and many leaves that sparkle in the sunshine and flutter in every breeze. It gives much shade and provides a fine resting place for travelers. It is an image of God, a joyful achievement. It is the product of a life of hammering by nature's hardships. Its quiet magnificence whispers the secret of life.

The privilege of having an old age such as this is given only to those who have lived macrobiotically.

Chapter 9

Sickness

The Most Difficult Disease

I have almost never met an illness that has resisted cure by way of macrobiotics — its healing power has amazed me time and again. All patients become well, and especially those who are most seriously ill.

After thirty years of experience, however, I recognize one ailment as being truly unique and difficult to handle. It is one from which *most* people suffer.

If this ailment is not overcome completely, the patient is always a potential victim — he becomes ill again and again. In this sense it is like the tapeworm that plagues most Japanese, but it does infinitely more damage.

Western medicine cannot cure the basic condition that enables the tapeworm to develop; it only prescribes a medicine that expels it. Sooner or later the worm returns. More medicine is then administered and the cycle repeats itself. After having been used once, twice, five times, the medicine no longer works; the dosage must be increased. Too much of it, however, and blindness is the result.

Macrobiotics eliminates this condition in just a couple of weeks. Either the worm is regurgitated or expelled through the bowels.

Recently a young boy vomited a cupful of tapeworms five days after starting macrobiotics. At first he thought that he had brought up noodles but changed his mind when they moved. Since then, he has not been able to pass a noodle shop without getting ill.

Although macrobiotics can eliminate tapeworms, dropped stomach (gastroptosis), tuberculosis, asthma, pneumonia, diabetes, and kidney illness very easily, the ailment that I spoke of earlier is harder to deal with.

Not too long ago, I sent out about three hundred inquiries to people whom I had helped through my teaching. The inquiry included a stamped, addressed answer card printed as follows:

I have completely cured my sickness   ☐
I am partially cured   ☐
I have quit macrobiotics   ☐

The recipient of the card had only to check his answer and write in his name. After two months, I had received only 109 replies.

Here is the disease that plagues two out of three people — the most difficult of all maladies. Although it might be called idleness or stubbornness, it is nothing more than *arrogance*. Its victims know no gratitude or thankfulness; they miss the excitement and joy of living. They live a sad, dark life. They know no happiness — only coldness and living death. They always complain and give nothing but trouble to others. Even a dog expresses joy when he sees a friend or his master, but these people *never* emerge from the darkness. They become sick again and again, and usually die early.

I was once consulted by a woman who had been suffering for ten years. Macrobiotics gave her the help she had not found anywhere else. One year later she came back to see me and said, "I have forgotten my sickness since my consultation with you. I have forgotten what sickness is. My suffering has disappeared completely."

The fact that after her recovery she did do her best to teach others the method that had cured her reveals at least a bit of gratitude. The average person never returns or expresses thanks. He forgets about everything as soon as his pain is gone.

Those who know true gratefulness *never* forget that they were once ill; they always remember who or what healed them and are eternally thankful.

The most difficult person to cure is the arrogant one. He is the egoist who knows no joy and who does not mind bothering others as long as his needs are satisfied, the man who lives but has no real life.

Unless we cure this fundamental illness, it is useless to consider anything else that might trouble a patient, for such a person can never be happy. If I cannot change him, I have no right to teach macrobiotics; better that I give it up. Many people think to themselves, "I am healthy," or "I understand." They are the worst offenders — the sickest; the man who is *certain* that he is wise is actually the stupidest.

Macrobiotics can be summed up as the way that gives happiness and thus cures such arrogance. This, not the elimination of specific disease, is our aim.

Everybody is healthy; if not, it is his own crime.

The Healing Power of the Mind

I am convinced that a sick man is a criminal and that sickness is his punishment. Small children are exceptions since they are not old enough to judge for themselves. Their punishment is meted out instead to their parents in the form of the anguish they suffer when the children are ill.

Anyone who becomes ill or has ailing children knows neither God nor the Order of the Universe.

Our bodies — knowable, seeable, touchable — are part of and bound to this relative, material world. Our minds, by contrast, are absolutely free to go anywhere at any time in the absolute, infinite world. We have the power to look into the past or future in an instant.

The world of mind is in reality the world of God; it is Infinity or Oneness. Since all of us possess a mind, we are inhabitants without choice of the absolute world of God. We cannot say, in all honesty, that we do not know it. He who says, "I do not know God," or who behaves as if he does not know Him, is the biggest criminal of all. Compared with him, all other offenders are petty.

He who cannot live in the infinite world — the world of mind — will never be happy or achieve anything of real worth. He always ends in sickness and sorrow.

Epictetus has said, "Of all the things to be known, there is only one that is worth classifying as either *good* or *bad*. To know or acknowledge God or Infinity is a *good* thing. Not to know or acknowledge either one is *bad*. The consideration of good or bad in reference to all other things is by comparison insignificant and inconsequential." It is the product of a superficial concept of the world.

In macrobiotics we say that sickness comes from food. This can be proven to be true. Our *choice* of food, however, is actually determined by the mind. If we know God, or Mind, we never choose bad food. He who does not know God and cannot see the Order of the Universe cannot find the right food and becomes sick.

Physical illness is an indication of illness of mind or illness in thinking.

Mind and God being one and the same, it is easy to see that what overcomes illness is Mind. If one does not enter this world of Mind, one can neither cure disease nor be happy. In the Orient, mind means *absolute* or *Tao* or *discipline*. In this light it is understandable that for God it is not difficult to cure sickness and unhappiness.

Since in macrobiotics we understand that sickness of character or mind is caused by food, we naturally feel that its cure as well is rooted in food. From this fundamental point, it is a simple thing to eliminate physical illness.

He who thinks that macrobiotics is merely a cure for physical ailments, however, can never really be helped. It is not a new medicine to stop pain or suffering, but rather a teaching that goes to the *source* of pain and eradicates it. Once this kind of cure has been effected, the disease will never recur. Consequently, macrobiotic consultation is given once in a lifetime. I consult with an individual one time; those who return again indicate that they have never sought out the true cause of their difficulty.

Some people think that macrobiotics is no more than the teaching of a diet — the eating of gomasio, carrots, and brown rice. Others imagine that it is summed up in the statement, "Don't eat cake and sugar." How far from the truth!

Macrobiotics is the process of changing ourselves so that we can eat anything we like without fear of becoming ill; it enables us to live a joyful life during which we can achieve anything we choose. It is knowing the Infinite, living in the Infinite, giving thanks to the Infinite and always having a feeling of wonder and gratefulness towards the Infinite. Without this we do not have real health; our lives are spent in the contemplation of suffering and trouble.

Should an individual happen to have physical health alone, without being on intimate terms with the Infinite, he will never feel great joy or security. If he observes the macrobiotic way of life, however, he will inevitably acquire the mentality with which to live a happy life, in peace always.

The person who has never been sick is not truly secure because his health is a gift from his parents. They have provided him with a strong foundation that he can eventually destroy through bad judgment.

True health is that which you yourself have created out of illness. Only if you have produced your own health can you know how wonderful it actually is. For this reason, many healthy people squander away their health; through ignorance they spoil it without knowing its true value. He who knows the real worth of health spreads his joyous knowledge by telling others what he knows. If you are healthy but do not try to give to others of the happiness it brings, you are unaware that happiness is priceless.

The aim of macrobiotics is to provide the means for establishing a joyful attitude. In the face of it, all arrogance, complaints, fear, insecurity, sadness, and suffering fade into nothingness. Happiness, love, freedom, and belief remain. In such a state there is infinite gratitude.

We give thanks to and for everything. The man who is at this level radiates gratitude; his world is full. Even if he becomes ill or has great difficulty, such a man can change his suffering into happiness immediately. If someone attacks him with a stone, that stone changes into a flower; if the weapon is a sword, the sword becomes a mirror. If he is given poison, the poison is medicine.

Macrobiotics teaches us to translate this ephemeral, narrow, relative, sad, unfree world into an infinitely joyful heaven.

If you have neither the intention to understand nor the desire to enter this Seventh Heaven, you had better not be macrobiotic. He who does not want to enter Seventh Heaven has the biggest sickness of all — egotism. He is no better than those who seek only fame, wealth or position. Here is the biggest crime — the foundation of all unhappiness. What greater unhappiness can there be than to think, "Now I am rich" or "I have nothing to worry about — I am healthy." Wealth or health of this variety can change to poverty or sickness overnight.

Macrobiotics is as necessary for healthy people as it is for the sick; in fact, the so-called healthy ones must be helped first. But since they are usually content with their small good fortune and are not seeking anything more, they are difficult to reach. People who are suffering are easily helped because they have a reason to seek health — pain.

He who is sick and still understands Infinity is much happier than he who is healthy but cannot enter Seventh Heaven. I am thus grateful for illness.

Western medicine cures the symptoms of illness by artificial means such as an injection or a pill; the patient's understanding never enters into the whole process. Those treated in this manner lose their chance to enter the Kingdom of Heaven. I believe that Western medicine does man a great injustice in this way.

Healing power is in our minds. The material for opening our minds and for healing disease, however, is *food*, the qualities of which we distinguish through our minds. If we cannot clear our minds, we cannot distinguish correct food. *Healing power is in the mind.* Sickness is given to us so that we may discover this mind. If we cannot, we had better remain ill until we do. This is the order of God.

We must be grateful to Western medicine. Through the suffering it gives us, we have the motivation to change, to understand God and the Order of the Universe. We are thus given the opportunity to achieve the fullest health and happiness.

Thankfulness for Sickness

> "Behold the fowl of the air, for they sow not, neither do they reap, nor gather into barns. Yet, your Heavenly Father feedeth them. Are ye not better than they?"
>
> (Matthew 6:26)

Our search for health and longevity begins either when we fall ill or after we reach the age of forty and begin feeling weakness. Thus sickness and weakness are necessary in this world. It is through our efforts to change them into health that we learn gratitude. How dull life would be without the challenge they present!

A great scholar named Toju Nakae, the Saint of Ohmi (a province near Kyoto, Japan), was scolded often by his mother during his youth. He usually accepted the scolding obediently, without protest or complaint. On one particular occasion, however, he burst into tears. "Why do you cry?" his surprised mother asked. "Because your scolding has become weak," he replied. "It tells me that you are getting old and I am very sad."

The parents of this sort of child have much cause for happiness — he will be an important man as a direct result of the strict discipline with which he has been raised.

Scolding by our parents is part of our training for life and we should look up to them with gratitude for it. Either we get this training from them when we are young or from life itself later on; we can not escape it, nor should we try. By the same token, we should not attempt to side-step the scolding of God — sickness. It is this punishment that causes our minds to seek Him out.

To overcome sickness by means of injections or operations is to evade God's punishment or scolding. Just as we should be sad if our parents have died and there is no one to scold us, so should we be sad if we do not get sick. We must be grateful for it; if we hate it, we reveal our egotism and cowardice.

We must accept everything given by God with pleasure, including sickness. In winter we must enjoy cold, in summer heat. Animals in their natural environment accept nature as it is without using artificial means to change it; as a result they are healthier than men. Man in his search for pleasure and comfort finds only weakness and disease. To forsake artificial civilization and *return to nature* is to find the macrobiotic way of life.

This Second World War will continue for longer than we expect with the result that the necessities for living — food, clothing, housing — will become very scarce. Our food supply will dwindle to less than one-third of what it is now, as happened to the Germans during the First World War. Furthermore, this scarcity will make prices go up. At that time it will be easy to be macrobiotic because there will be less food of all kinds, particularly expensive ones.[9] We will be limited to grains and thus have a good opportunity to practice the macrobiotic way of living. Whoever observes macrobiotics has no need to worry about food problems. He will be as free as the birds in the sky.

The following statement was made by the Meiji Emperor of Japan, conqueror of both Russia and China:

Rather than take medicine when I am ill,
I prefer to take righteous food every day.

Japan was very macrobiotic during his reign. It was at this time that Admiral Perry opened the Orient to the West. The Emperor was a man of wide interests guided by a deep sense of order. He felt that certain things did not merit being placed high on the scale of values. Contrast this with the Japan of today where the worst is accepted as being on the same level as the best.

Since the time when I cured my own illness with macrobiotics twenty years ago, I have never been sick. If I have suffered, I have been very thankful. For instance, I once hurt both my heels and the pain lasted for sixty days but I applied no treatment.

This year I developed a sore throat after staying too long in a warm, heated room. I took no treatment because this suffering was a warning that let me know that my body had become weakened. As long as I am suffering, I am careful with my eating and drinking habits. For this very reason I avoid treatments. Surely you see that with this attitude, even if you have a sickness, you are not really sick.

It is more important to reach a similar level of understanding or state of mind than it is to learn to apply any treatment, no matter how effective.

Rigidity

In your attempt to practice macrobiotics, you may encounter many difficulties. A place to buy the food may not be readily available; if you find the place to buy, the price may be too high; your family, friends, community, society or the whole world may be against the idea.

In any event, do not worry. The first task that faces you is this one: *understand the principle*. You can then apply it no matter what the difficulties may be.

Animals, birds, and flowers live macrobiotically without money. Study and think about them and their lives, about primitive peoples, about the experiences of Robinson Crusoe. Look at the world around you; there are innumerable sources of encouragement and hope upon which to draw.

If you have allowed yourself to believe that your illness is incurable, that there is no hope left, you will not be able to summon up the energy for such investigation and work. Your drive is gone. You are defeated, you have conceded the victory, you have given up the ship; you had better stop living. Even if you live a long life under such circumstances, you will be half asleep anyhow. Human life is not much when compared with the universe, and we did not come here by our own will, so why cling to it so hard? No matter how long we live we must die sometime; we all leave this world eventually. We are only passengers on an express train called Earth, and when we reach our destination, we must disembark.

For those who follow macrobiotics, it is not much different. Suppose they manage to live for one hundred years; that length of time, too, is only a second compared to the life of the universe.

Achieve this kind of understanding and free your rigid mind. Then you can *live*. Without a free mind you die very quickly. With it you can study and think. You will have something to do. And with something to do in this world we can live; with nothing to do we die. Idleness is a killer.

The individual who no longer has a rigid mind has found freedom. He has given up his vice-like grip on his own mind; he has given up the prerogative, the illusion that there is a freedom of choice; he does not care whether or not his mind is his own; *he can freely accept the decisions of nature.*

Life can be so easy. Refuse to let go and you are a person drowning; the more you struggle, the faster you sink.

Nature . . . she brought us into being, she has nurtured us. We are obligated to humbly and gratefully obey her. When it is time to die, we die. If it is not our time, nature will preserve us by showing us the way.

Whoever cannot be macrobiotic because of poverty is very fortunate and has cause for much happiness. Difficulties of any kind will make him the happiest of all men because he will have more to be grateful for when he finally does become macrobiotic. He who is able to be macrobiotic with ease cannot know gratefulness. The poor person is grateful for a penny. The millionaire is never grateful; even a gift of one thousand dollars leaves him unimpressed. So, he who has more difficulties is more happy. His gratitude makes him happy and healthy.

He who says, "I cannot practice macrobiotics" does not understand it fully. But suppose that we observe macrobiotics to the letter, repeating everything that we have heard like a phonograph. We are still not macrobiotic. We must reach the point where we can eat *anything* without fear of losing our health and happiness. We must control our lives by ourselves. If we adhere to a diet that has been devised by someone else, our lives are not our own. *We must not be rigid.* Here is a striking example of what I mean:

A mother once came to me for some advice regarding her sick son. I suggested a diet for him to follow and he recovered his health. Years later I met him again — a small, very tense boy of dark complexion. I inquired as to what he had been eating. His mother replied that she still fed him the very yang (contractive, rich in sodium) diet that I had prescribed six years earlier when he was ill. Although he had been healthy for most of the six years that I had not seen him, she had mechanically continued to feed him food designed for an invalid! The result was that this boy became over-yang. He looked just like the *kinpira* (sliced, sauteed carrots and burdock root) that he had been eating for six years — small, dried-out, shrivelled. This is the end result of macrobiotics that has been mechanically applied with no knowledge or understanding of the basic principle involved.

Great difficulties arise when one's mate or parents are

against macrobiotics. If, however, you are humble they will soon yield and accept your way. If your husband is against macrobiotics, your attitude is wrong and you do not love him enough. *You love your ego more.*

Another woman came to me with the following story:

"My husband doesn't allow macrobiotics in our home. He gives our children meat and candy. What's more, he keeps another woman, a professional. He contracted a disease and passed it on to me. That is why I have tried to start macrobiotics but he has never permitted it. As soon as I cure one sickness, he brings home another because he changes girls so often. I have been living such a life for twenty years. What should I do? Where shall I turn? Sometimes I have thought of suicide but I cannot bring myself to it . . . we have five children and another on the way. I can't go home to my parents because I am so ashamed; furthermore, they will not accept my return because tradition in our country does not permit it. I don't care for myself but I am very worried about my children. Worst of all, my husband has had an affair with my youngest sister. I know it because she is both ill and pregnant. Life is hell. Yesterday I asked him to please confine himself to one mistress. He told me to be quiet, that he would decide what to do for himself. I asked him to at least be careful and keep himself free of disease. He said, 'I am a professional soldier. How can I be so cowardly as to worry about disease?' Then he hit me. What should I do? Where shall I turn?"

I have heard many cases such as this — at least six this year alone. Generally, they involve the wives of educators and doctors, rarely those of businessmen. All these women seem to have the same weakness . . . they have all been eating bad food with the result that they are ill, either physically or mentally. That is why their husbands are not satisfied and look elsewhere. They give no joy and inspire no confidence; their husbands consequently refuse them most anything including the freedom to follow macrobiotics. These women seldom realize that all their difficulties are of their own making.

When I explain this to them, they understand quickly and with great joy. As a result their families have become much happier and their husbands more gentle than ever before. The discovery of the *primary* cause of their difficulties produces miracles.

I cannot change the mentality of a woman but I can help her to change her physiology through macrobiotics. If her physiology changes, she becomes healthy and enjoys her work; she is more efficient and more happy. Her husband and family reflect this happiness.

In a case where the bulk of the trouble lies with the husband, it is easy to overcome because the wife controls the kitchen. She determines what her mate is like by what she feeds him.

The greatest difficulty arises when the wife is against macrobiotics. No matter how hard the husband tries, it is almost hopeless. For example, twenty years ago I told a friend about macrobiotics but his wife was dead-set against it and he died soon after.

A wife who refuses to even try macrobiotics will eventually destroy both her husband and her family; she is a detriment to society. A man had better divorce such a wife as soon as possible for time will not change her mind. Her husband will have perished long before that happens.

Confucius said, "Women and small-minded men are hard to control." I feel very sad for him — his wife must have been very difficult to get along with. The wife who does not understand and accept macrobiotics makes it difficult for her family and herself to avoid an unhappy end.

Without a basic principle to follow, any sort of practice is no more than superstition. The principle and spirit of macrobiotics lie in the recognition, experiencing, and understanding of nature. This is *Tao* — the return to and contemplation of God.

Chapter 10

The Secret Medicine

Severe tuberculosis eliminated in two months by Mr. Wago; a thirty-year-old case of leprosy overcome by Mr. Tsutsumi; colitis cured by General Matsui in three weeks; a combination of asthma and skin disease that had lasted for *forty years* gone in one month; cancer of the womb, cancer of the breast, rheumatism, arthritis, poliomyelitis, female baldness and infertility, the inability to speak, tuberculosis of the spine and kidney . . . I have been witnessing the disappearance of these and many other diseases for over twenty years in those individuals who have deeply understood natural living.

The thought of all the people who have been saved by macrobiotics in the past, plus the fact that I too was rescued from certain death over twenty years ago, makes me feel nothing less than endless gratitude and thankfulness every day.

Experience has shown me that the more severe the illness, the shorter the cure. A slight illness is more difficult only because the patient does not take his problem too seriously.

A very few people, possibly one in ten, do not respond in the usual four to eight weeks. They have come to macrobiotics too late and unfortunately cannot be helped. They have waited much too long before seeking help and are regrettably destined to die.

It is usually so easy to help the sick that I am amazed when I think about it. I then wonder why so many people (including myself) fall ill in the first place, why they tolerate suffering for so long.

The answer is a simple one: we are all ignorant of the simple, clear relationship between food and life. Anyone who understands this basic teaching of macrobiotics knows how foolish it is to become ill; with such knowledge he can be sick no more. Yet at times I think that it would be fun to be sick once again because it has been over twenty years since I suffered last!

In macrobiotics we never use medicine; our pharmacy is the kitchen. Our method is based on the potency of daily food —simple things like brown rice, carrots, onions, radishes, burdock root, miso and sea vegetables.

How such commonplace foods can affect so many strange ailments and eliminate them in one or two months is very puzzling to people with a scientific orientation. "Why do so many desperately weakened victims thrive on it?" they ask. "What is the secret?"

When a man falls ill, his friends offer the usual sympathetic advice. "Take it easy, eat some good food, rest . . ."

But illness is not a precious jewel. If we nurture it, we preserve it for a long time. The disease — *not the human being* — must be thrown away like the useless thing that it is.

In theory, we all know that we live because we eat. Not one of us, however, seems to have a practical answer to the important questions:

> What is the right food?
> What is the right quantity?
> What is the right method of preparation?
> What is the right manner in which to eat?

Given the right food, we can live a happy, healthy, peaceful life. Given food that is *not* right, we are no longer right men —we are inhuman beings. We become weak, sick, poor, incapable of working — joyless.

What then is right food?

If our approach is analytical, this is a very difficult question to answer. Protein, fats, carbohydrates, vitamins, minerals, calories — so many things to consider. No one as yet has given a concrete, livable answer to our question in this way, not even scientists, scholars, and specialists.

Take protein, for instance. Are there two experts who agree about the kind and quantity needed by human beings?

Vitamins and minerals are in the same category. People say, "Apples are good for you." But who tells us how many ounces to eat, when to eat them, and how to prepare an apple properly so that it is fit for us to consume?

I know of one boy who ate too many apples and eventually died of children's dysentery. An elementary school teacher died after eating thirty-two apples in four days on the advice of her physician. One famous doctor of nutrition, a great believer in the effectiveness of apples, died recently from an excess of them. I could go on and on — the list of casualties from food abuse is a very long one.

There obviously is a right amount for everything. "Too much of even a good thing is not wise." But who knows what is too much?

Vitamin C is supposedly very important for good nutrition. How much and how often? Since no two people have the same constitution or character, since everyone's physical condition is different, can we establish a standard amount that would be practical in every situation? We suspect that whoever seeks this answer is running a fool's errand.

But what if by some strange miracle the experts were able to determine the right amount? Some nations might not be capable of producing enough of it to supply an entire population. Some places could not store enough for everyone. And many individuals could not afford the price of their basic needs.

It is so difficult to apply such a theory practically and even theoretically. There must be a simpler way.

Throughout history, men have lived happy lives without complicated analytical concepts of nutrition. Although our ancestors gave little thought to apples, they were healthier, happier, and wiser than we are. Even beasts seem to be able to live joyfully without concerning themselves with chemistry or scientific detail. Perhaps there is hope for us too.

We are so far removed from simplicity! We hear and read things like this: "Lack of scientific information and illness go hand-in-hand." "Health is the result of research; research costs money; money is therefore essential to health."

But what about the millions of people in the history of the

world who led full lives long before science became so important, and on much less money than we spend today?

"Animal protein and calcium are basic to good nutrition." Isn't it curious that a cow can produce not only the meat and milk that we feel is so essential for us but her own massive bone structure as well from a diet of grasses alone?

If the modern, superstitious belief in science, money, and meat is a valid one, how miserable we are. A poor man is forever excluded — he can neither be healthy nor enjoy his life. Existence is no more than a game of chance in which the cards are stacked in favor of the rich, the educated, the knowledgeable.

It cannot be that God would create anything so unfair. *Anybody* can live joyfully in health.

If we compare the food that we eat today with that of our ancestors, we are struck by the vast difference between the two. So important a staple as rice was once cultivated with natural fertilizers while today the laboratory supplies them. We begin to suspect that the big problem lies in the area of what is natural and what is unnatural.

Few of us question the fact that it is natural for man to be born, to be active, to grow. And we agree that it is natural to depend upon food for life and survival. At this point, however, we fail to see the obvious.

Of all things that grow on a farm, the strongest seem to be the natural grasses — the weeds. The farmer easily spends as much time and effort eliminating them as he does cultivating his produce — and still they grow again and again naturally, by themselves, in the face of every chemical obstacle. Any farmer who has battled weeds will agree that they are more resistant than anything he grows for human consumption.

Here is the clue to successful existence. The ingenuity of science is juvenile as compared to the quietly irresistible force with which nature animates the entire universe.

> To live and be active, man depends upon food;
> To live naturally, he must eat natural foods;
> If he lives naturally, a man can be healthy and happy.

Since man is a natural product of a natural environment, he

must live as close to nature as possible; to be healthy and happy he must eat natural foods. This is the secret of macrobiotics.

But what are natural foods? They are the ones that our ancestors have used for a thousand years. And they differ from one country and climate to the next. This is why there are so many nationalities, religions, societies, and customs.

What was most natural for Japan, for example, was determined long ago through experience over countless generations; it consisted of over 800 foods that grew on mountains, in the sea, in rivers and fields. (This is the largest variety in use by any country in the world. France has but 300, Mongolia a mere five!) And they are still available today — one has only to look.

The Japanese diet was originally divided into two separate categories — principal foods and secondary ones. Evidence of such early awareness of the importance of food and value of some kinds of nourishment over others is not found in the culture of any other country.

The Japanese language as well reflects a similar depth of understanding. *Gohan,* the word for eating, refers to the taking of principal (not secondary) food. It symbolizes all eating but specifically pertains to whole rice. In the broadest sense, it means *grain.*

In traditional Japan, rice — principal food — was called the *God of toyo-uke.* (*Toyo-uke* means "receive plenty.") It was understood that a man became one with the Infinite by eating rice. It was the source of life, the materialization of God. It was accorded the highest respect and enshrined as a national symbol.

I agree that to follow any teaching blindly, even that of our ancestors, is unwise. Merely to eat as we have been taught is not enough. But to reject that teaching without trying to understand it is equally foolish. The result is what we have today; the keen insight of our ancestors has been completely forgotten. It lies ignored, discarded as old-fashioned.

One might say that macrobiotics is the teaching that is rooted in the concept of principal food. It is a reaffirmation and reapplication of the ancient wisdom and has produced the miraculous results that lead to an inevitable conclusion: *we must re-evaluate, relearn, and apply the concept of principal food in our daily lives.* We must know that food is important and know the reasons why it is vital to our present and future well-being. Otherwise, we are unqualified to be healthy, happy, and peaceful.

This is the secret of macrobiotics.

Chapter 11

Truth Is Simple

That which is simple:
   wholeness and nature

That which is complicated:
   the parts of the whole
   those things that are human or produced by man
   thinking
   activity

Leaves of grass — green, simple, beautiful, natural — shapes endless in variety yet never strange, unfamiliar, or artificial . . .

No one can duplicate this naturalness. We can analyze its parts, imitate its color or form; but its vitality, its physiological and chemical activity, its power to grow — all of this eludes us. Human understanding cannot encompass it.

There is no factory in existence that can remove carbon dioxide from the air, produce its own oxygen, and then change the whole thing into carbohydrate with the addition of a little sunshine. Yet this complex process occurs simply and with little effort in a blade of grass.

A tree — fifty or even seventy feet tall with roots that go deep into the earth; branches that reach out in every direction, that bow to the ground in the grip of a storm and then spring back to their former shape and position with the ceasing of the wind. Rain is its sweet bath, snow its wrap of ermine. No complaint or protest — it gratefully accepts both good and bad.

Seen at a distance in its totality, the tree that has stood for a hundred years or more is a thing of natural beauty. It is so simple. If we approach more closely, if we examine its detail under a microscope or analyze it chemically, we find a complex miracle forever beyond our comprehension.

The living human, God's natural product, has a deceptively simple exterior: two arms, two legs, a torso, a head. But examine them closely — what complexity! A hand consists of only one palm and five fingers, but its wonderful power has made history through an endless variety of acts, both virtuous and criminal. This seemingly elementary tool has produced all of civilization.

Biologists and anatomists have found what they have labelled heart, lungs, nerves, and intestines — small, quiet mechanisms covered by skin. The life that causes them to function, however, is a complexity that resists analysis.

And what of memory? We easily remember things that have happened thirty or forty years in the past and enjoy singing songs learned in childhood. What device can record, file away, and instantaneously replay memories from so long ago? Perhaps someone will eventually construct one but it will be far more complicated than our human function, just as the finest camera cannot compare with the complex simplicity of the human eye.

Human productivity always appears complex on its surface. A house, an airplane, a watch, a radio — each is a mass of detail that proves to be very simple upon close scrutiny.

Health or true life, a natural state of being for living things, is simple. It is soundless — no motor runs so quietly. When we attempt to discover and analyze all its details, however, we undertake the same impossibly useless task we faced in probing the mysteries of the blade of grass or the tree.

We had best do the only thing that we can; give in, accept this wonderful gift of nature and enjoy it. We must give thanks and live happily and joyfully. We can do no more.

The apparent simplicity of nature that is revealed to be infinite complication itself requires only earth, sunshine, wind and water for full existence. A man needs no more to be assured a joyous life.

In the morning he awakens easily to find that he has visitors — a breeze that is the breath of God, sunshine that is the glance of the Mother of Life. He eats naturally — grains, seeds, leaves, roots, grasses in all forms. He adds a few grains of salt — a reminder of his briny origin. This and some clear spring water. Nothing more. How simple and uncomplicated a breakfast table!

Macrobiotic cuisine has the taste of the primitive, the flavor of *haiku*[10] and the tea ceremony. Its final product is simplicity itself yet it holds infinite complexity within. It has the taste of nature. He who cannot distinguish it from that of the artificial, elaborate food found in restaurants and supermarkets will spend a sad life because he is caught in a web of artificiality. He will surely spoil his health and end tragically.

Of late, many people have become enthusiastic about hiking, mountain-climbing, skiing, and camping. Most of them are trying to find or maintain health through some kind of contact with nature; they seek her out with a vengeance. Meanwhile, their rucksacks are bursting with chocolate, candy, wine, butter, fruit, canned goods, ham, sausage — all *artificial foods*. It is hard for me to understand how they can devote themselves so energetically to the pursuit of nature and still bring such unnatural foodstuffs into her presence. It is like working long hours to buy a plane ticket to Tokyo and then blindly boarding the plane that flies in the opposite direction.

Natural food is so very important because it is the condensation or crystallization of sunshine, air, and water — the source of life. Sunshine, air, and water are not too difficult to find in their original forms but the search for natural food involves problems.

Most of what we eat today comes to us from remote places; it grows in one season and we use it during another. It is consequently frozen and/or artificially preserved in order to be salable. Even those things that are produced in nearer places have been grown with chemical fertilizers and insecticides to protect them and stimulate growth. They are all unnatural foods.

The majority of the fish eaten in the Tokyo area comes from foreign places like the South China Sea, the Gulf of Mexico, and the South Pacific. They travel a distance of at least 1500 miles to reach the consumer.

The same is true for fruit. It grows far from the consumer and is the product of a season other than the one in which it is used. If it reaches the market in winter, it is summer produce; if used in the spring, it grew in the fall.

All fruits today are grown with strong insecticides and chemical fertilizers that are harmful to human beings and are inevitably poisonous. They are unnaturally cultivated products that are far removed from what nature intended as is indicated by their lack of flavor, their exaggerated size, and their excessive potassium content.

Commercially prepared cakes are no different. They are made with tropical sugar grown 1500 miles away and chocolate that originates at a distance of 4000 miles. They contain artificial coloring and preservatives that, while they do not kill a man instantaneously, will wear him away in time.

To eat such foods is to commit slow suicide. To produce them is to be guilty of slow murder.

Saints and wise men have long advised, "Return to nature." And because they have been so abstract and mystical about the means whereby this is achieved, it has been the rare individual who has succeeded in living by their words.

Some have tried forsaking the conveniences of the civilized world — cars, radio, telephones, steam heat — and have only changed the external, superficial part of their lives. Even if we live like our animal cousins — unshaven, unwashed, unclad, sleeping on a bed of pine needles with a blanket of leaves as our cover — nature eludes us.

Yet the method that makes a return to nature possible is so very simple. There is no other way than by making ourselves, our organisms, *one* with her. We must eat natural foods.

The world of life is governed by the law of God: *the body and the land are not two.* Whoever ignores this suffers just punishment — sickness, deterioration, degeneration — because he cannot adapt to his surroundings. Neither individuals, nor races, nor man as a whole are exempt.

The healthy, happy man has understood that to live a joyful life, no matter where on this earth, he must first of all make himself one with his environment. He must eat, drink, and behave in a manner that does not alienate him from the orderly, simple truth of nature.

He must discover natural food — that which grows in his immediate area — uncontaminated by the imposed, artificial protection that science misguidedly offers through insecticides, pesticides, artificial fertilizers, preservatives, and additives.

If we want to live in this world — so joyful and yet so severe because it offers no way out of the punishment that is dealt out to those who swim against the current of life, the orderliness of the universe — we must look to and never forget nature.

In our material world, two viewpoints exist side by side, again reminding us that yin and yang are ever present everywhere.

The mechanical, analytical, scientific viewpoint sees all things as separate — separated from themselves, separate from men. Not only are they apart from man, in this sense, but they are created to be subservient to him, subject to his every whim.

With this as justification, men arrogantly impose themselves upon one another and their surroundings in a vain effort to find happiness, health, and peace. The end result is disease, tragedy, and war.

The *spiritual* viewpoint that originates in Seventh Heaven or Infinity sees *all* things as being one. Nature is God; God is Truth; Truth is the eternal order that simplifies infinite complexity to the greatest degree.

If you comprehend this, you are a poet. Your understanding of the consummate beauty of nature is such that your life itself becomes poetry. And all that you write is poetic without your having set out to make it so.

Everyone without exception has the right to know Truth. For that very reason, Truth has the responsibility to be uncomplicated — simple. For the same reason, the principle of life and health — macrobiotics, the nutritional path to longevity — is Truth because it is so simple.

Health — not merely the absence of disease, but the dynamic balance that nature maintains so effortlessly — is a usual state of being in the universe. It is natural and simple; it is identical with order; it cannot be produced artificially with machines or pills, science notwithstanding.

If health is natural, what could be more fitting and orderly than to achieve a state of well-being by following the simple way of nature?

Intuitively, without material proof being necessary, we know that nature or God or the Whole exists. Our spirit, our soul, our mind intuits or recognizes it by a method that is beyond logic, a way that is superlogical. In reality, intuition is the manifestation of Wholeness itself.

Our human body is part of the Whole. It owes its very existence to it. The Whole is nature and Whole Nature is our spirit.

To know God, to recall nature, to acknowledge Wholeness is the highest wisdom to which a human being can aspire. The highest form of discipline with which to achieve such wisdom is the macrobiotic way of living.

Chapter 12

No Incurable Disease

Belief

No matter what method we use in the attempt to overcome sickness, we must first of all have a strong *will to cure*. This is particularly true for the macrobiotic way since here the individual must cure himself by himself and for himself, through his own comprehension of what is the true cause of his suffering.

We must be filled with the belief that our sickness can and will be cured through macrobiotics. This is neither a rigid, mystical, religious, unfounded belief nor a blind superstition. It is, rather, deepest understanding — the realization that justifiably and by all that is right, macrobiotics *should* cure illness for us because it has done just that for thousands of years in the Orient. It has simply and practically taught what is righteous food and natural living. It has inevitably led towards health, beauty, wisdom, and happiness.

I do not say dogmatically that those who believe in macrobiotics will be cured while the nonbelievers will suffer. I merely say that if it is not too late for a real cure, macrobiotics will achieve one because it is the way of nature.

I believe that illness is the crystallization of an error in our judgment, the tangible sign of a lack of natural orderliness in our lives.

In allowing this condition to arise, either through poor thinking, ignorance, or apathy, we have done something wrong. To be healthy again, we must make a change — we must do something right. We must re-establish the orderly kind of existence that underlies and guarantees health.

By becoming macrobiotic you undertake the rewarding task of putting your life in order, starting from its most basic point — eating and drinking. As a consequence, God will release you from all sickness. In the same manner, a man who has been unjustly accused of a crime will eventually be freed simply because it is *right* and *just* that he be freed. To see this clearly and distinctly is to know what it is that constitutes true belief.

Righteous food is the materialization of God. He is revealed to us in it and by means of it. Our body — converted food — thus constitutes a speck of God Himself. The very reason that we can even live in this universe is that we are a speck of Him. And the reason that this speck becomes sick or unhappy is that it forgets its origin; it loses sight of the totality of which it is a minute part.

If we know God or Wholeness and at the same time are deeply aware of our own personal *speckness*, we cannot avoid being beautiful, healthy, wise, and happy. To realize this and then to live with that realization as our motivation is macrobiotics.

Will

Will is vastly different from the impulse to escape from the symptoms of a disease, an urge prompted by pain and suffering. The person who seeks a palliative or pain-killer, who believes that his salvation lies in the right kind of surgery or in finding the right doctor, is motivated by short-sighted, wishful thinking — not will. True will is the relentless drive to discover the law of life — the origin, mechanism, structure, value, and end of Justice. If this is what stirs you to action, then all your ills are curable.

You must be able to say:

I *will* cure my sickness. I *will* live in Justice; I *will* live in God.

I am fearful and sick because I have violated the law of nature. To *discover* and *correct* this violation is more vital to my existence than the cure itself.

If I *understand* righteous macrobiotics — the materialization of the law of nature — my sickness must be cured.

If I cannot cure, then both my understanding and my way of making the law of nature a practical part of my life are superficial.

I must study more deeply.

This is *will*.

Physical Miracles

I believe in our miraculous bodies, in physical miracles that are beyond science and human knowledge, beyond explanation.

The first unicell that is conceived in a mother's womb becomes two, four, eight, one thousand, a million . . . it becomes a nervous system, stomach, intestine, lung, nose, hair skin, teeth. How wonderful!

Blood circulates, we move, sleep, eat, digest, the brain thinks, we speak — all miracles. As long as that which makes these things occur — the power of God or Life — is moving within us, we are *alive* and can cure sickness.

Mental Miracles

I believe in mental miracles and wonders.

About twenty years ago, I was employed by a trading company where Mr. Fukishima was my superior. I can never show enough respect for his memory because he has done me a great favor. Through him, I have had one of the most profound experiences of my life.

I vividly remember the time that he traveled to the South Pacific to negotiate a contract and left me in charge of the main office. I was so grateful for his faith in me that I worked from dawn to midnight every day, taking time out for only an occasional nap on the office table.

At midnight on September 30th, during a heavy rain, I lay napping and had the following dream:

I was at a pier in the port of Kobe. As I stood in the bright sunlight, a cargo train stopped in front of me. Its center door slid open noiselessly, revealing my superior clad in a white summer suit. "What has happened, Mr. Fukishima? You have returned so unexpectedly that your welcome party isn't even prepared."

I cannot describe the sensation I felt as I shook his hand. It was unbelievably cold. "What is the matter?" Tears rolled gently from his eyes and he smiled.

At that very instant my dream was broken by a knock at the office door. It was a telegraph messenger with a cable that read, "FUKISHIMA ILL STOP ADMITTED ARMY HOSPITAL SAIGON STOP." The following day I received notification that he had died.

I immediately packed my things and boarded an old French steamer, the S. S. Manchu, bound for South Vietnam. At noon ten days later I was in Mr. Fukishima's suite at the Hotel Rotunde.

Since offices, shops, and government agencies in Vietnam are customarily closed from noon to two o'clock, I decided to lie down a while to rest. I stretched out on the bed that Mr. Fukishima had occupied only a few days before and fell into an exhausted sleep.

An instant later, it seemed, Mr. Fukishima's voice woke me. My first impulse was to stand up but I could not move a muscle. I lay immobilized for an hour listening to him speak about me with Mr. Baba, my fellow employee.

His voice broke off abruptly at the sound of a loud knocking at the door. Only then did I manage to jump up from the bed. The room was empty.

I was so dazed by what had happened that it was some time before I realized that the knocking had not stopped. I ran to the door to find Mr. Baba.

In the next hour, he repeated exactly what I had heard from my bed earlier. His description of Mr. Fukishima's last moments of life completely unsettled me:

"Mr. Baba, I have just seen Mr. Ohsawa . . . " With that, Fukishima smiled and was no more.

All of what I had heard in the room — Mr. Fukishima's conversation — had apparently occurred at the time that I had seen him in my dream at our Japan office. He and I had both gone through the telepathic experience of seeing one another at the very same time.

* * *

Such mental or spiritual interplay is not new to me. I have experienced it several times in my life but especially since becoming macrobiotic. It happened again only recently.

On my return from Formosa, I visited the sickbed of my friend Mr. Natori and then boarded a Pullman train for Nigata. Soon after I had retired, Mr. Natori stood before me. "Ah, you have come to say good-bye. Don't worry, I will take care of everything," I said. He said nothing and disappeared.

Before my lecture the next day, I received a telegram from Tokyo. Mr. Natori had died at the very moment when he appeared before me on the train.

* * *

The human body, a minute part of the wholeness of the universe, is bound by time and space. The spirit, Wholeness itself, is not. It is free; it moves unfettered in dimensionless Infinity. Of this I am certain.

Our organism is comparable to a radio receiver; it can pick up the radio waves that fill the entire universe. What is even more miraculous is that we are transmitters as well. We can send messages to and from any place at any time provided that we are not bound by matter or body. Whenever we engage in real thinking or become purely spiritual, we de-limit our minds — we can transmit waves. At such times we possess a wonderful power.

The food that we eat can be likened to either the material out of which our receiver is constructed or the electricity that powers it. The quality and quantity of food that we take determines the amount of waves that our receiver-transmitter can pick up or send.

I accept this miracle and at the same time I want to know and understand it as deeply as possible. This is the way in which I live my life. If a healthy, long life were reflective of only the physical aspect of things, it would be an insignificant, pitifully sad yet troublesome consideration.

If, however, you delve so deeply into the spiritual world as to be able to use your physical body as a radio receiver, and if you live joyfully and happily as well, life is most wonderful. You can feel at times that you have lived a lifetime in no more than a few seconds.

The physical life is the false one. One hundred years of it are as nothing. It is the spiritual life that is real — one instant of it is priceless.

* * *

Let us make our bodies healthy with righteous food. We can thus enter into the miracles of the universe and enjoy a profound eternal life.

* * *

Regardless of whether we protect our body or abuse it, it will endure anywhere from forty to one hundred years. Good or bad on the physical level makes little difference.

To cure the body, to heal sickness, therefore, is not our aim. It is a worthless goal — it is *nothing*.

The important thing is joyfulness, happiness, and amusement in life from morning to night, from night to morning. A million dollars, a strong body, and/or social position are meaningless without them. The biggest, longest spiritual life — that is eternal.

* * *

Because the spirit is larger than the body, we can be happy in spite of illness. As difficult as it may seem to achieve, the ability to cure that illness is the certification that we know and understand the Order of Nature, the Law of God — the eternal, infinite world.

Essays

When Will You Be Cured?

A medical doctor wrote me a criticism after one summer camp:

> Regarding any criticism of yourself, professor, we are all trying our best to learn of Oriental philosophy and medicine. Whatever understanding or use we can and will make of your teachings, it must be realized that this will occur within the Occidental culture we live in; therefore, we must be dependent on criteria which are compatible with our circumstances. When we say a patient is completely cured, their circumstances of cure must be such that any physician would examine the patient and accept them as being in good health, not just mentally at peace and happy, but still evidencing on physical examination or lab examination the same findings which might have been originally present. It does not suffice to say that our method and techniques of examination are inadequate and inaccurate. Whatever errors they represent are constant and relative. I would like to see you more willing to interpret your opinions in terms that would satisfy our Occidental culture."

When will you be cured? I often answer, "You will be cured in ten days to two months." And yet you do not find yourself cured within that period. Why? I have stated repeatedly that macrobiotics cures all diseases within ten days, that it changes the body's orientation toward health, away from disease. Disease is the exact barometer of our mistakes, of our abuse, of our ignorance of the Order of the Universe. It is therefore said that there can be no cure unless we recognize our own faults, our own ignorance, and, above all, the Order of the Universe, the key to our health, freedom, and Justice. But what is Justice? Everyone thinks he knows, but in reality . . .

According to Oriental philosophy, Justice is absolute, infinite, eternal and universal — a larger concept, by far, than that of Western justice. The commonly understood meaning of justice is relative, personal, finite, and conditional. Democratic justice as defined by John Locke is only known by the majority. In actuality, there is no single concept in Western thought that is the equivalent of the Oriental concept of Justice. Justice is another name for happiness that is infinite and eternal. A macrobiotic individual is a student of the way to such infinite happiness. The Unique Principle or, in other words, life itself, is the only teacher of this all-embracing Justice.

Most of you look for a rapid cure, and make large statements about your willingness to pay any price to achieve it. Still, you only attempt to understand basic yin/yang functioning where it concerns your immediate diet. Worse yet, you allow others to tell you what to eat. You abandon all pursuit of the Unique Principle as soon as your physical difficulties have disappeared. In short, the patient is never willing to pay the true price.

Two persons come to mind, both of whom were not cured by macrobiotics. Each had been crippled for a long time previously. Neither could understand that disease cannot leave the patient until he discovers and acknowledges his own mistakes. So many individuals are relieved of their anxieties and suffering by following the macrobiotic diet, yet become ill again because they do not probe ever deeper into the Unique Principle, the Law of Life.

I have understood, once and for all, that one must not cure anyone. *Everyone must do it for himself, by himself.* If your wish is to gain a reputation, to have a good income, to enjoy a sentimental self-esteem, then you can, of course, make a career of taking care of people.

When will you be cured? In ten days, most assuredly, if you sincerely admit to yourself your own mistakes. The kind of disease makes no difference, since all diseases are a variation of man's loss of balance — biological, psychological, or spiritual. If you are not cured in ten days or two months, you have no right to criticize my teaching. You have only to regret your own poor understanding of infinite and absolute Justice.

Curing the Man

Macrobiotic practice can cure disease symptoms easily. The difficulty lies in curing the patient. He must learn how to unfetter himself, cast off his shackles, and walk upright, unafraid, a natural man, a free man. But learning to be free requires the total involvement of heart, imagination, faith, and will.

The technique to cure sickness is called medicine. To cure, one must know the cause of sickness. However, modern medicine does not know the cause. What modern medicine calls cause is merely *symptoms*, or the results of sickness. The reason modern medicine cannot cure so many diseases lies in the fact that it does not know the cause of disease.

Then what is the cause of disease? In my opinion, the cause of disease is the condition in which one's Supreme Judgment is clouded or eclipsed. All animals other than man have lower judgment only, which is the first, second and third stages of judgment, and are lacking the fourth, fifth, and sixth stages of judgment. Therefore, they reveal the Supreme Judgment more easily than man. In the case of man, who has the fourth through sixth stages of judgment, the Supreme Judgment is eclipsed. But why do the fourth, fifth, and sixth stages of judgment eclipse the seventh stage or Supreme Judgment?

Judgment is a compass giving us directions and decisions in our travels through life. One who makes a wrong judgment goes the wrong direction, and the result is unhappiness or sickness. Sickness is the first warning that we have made a wrong judgment. A healthy person never is unhappy. If he is, his health is only physical, not total and real health; or his health is "given" health from parents or others.

For example, we may analyze a painting by the amount, quality, and cost of color used. But by improving these, we can never improve the picture. The skill of the painter must be improved. For that, his thinking, idea, or concept of life must be improved. Modern medicine tries to cure sickness by analyzing the color. It is forgetting the painter completely, who uses the color and designs the picture.

Most medicine aims at curing symptoms. When it realizes that the symptomatic cure is useless or endless or dangerous, it turns to other ways. One of them is psychic, psychological, and religious healing, and the other one is social and preventive medicine. However, these tend to be symptomatic cures. Macrobiotic medicine aims at curing man, and not sickness only, because man is the producer of sickness. Without curing man, no sickness is cured.

Western medicine must develop to be a preventive medicine. Preventive medicine must develop into the way of health — macrobiotics. The way of health must reach to a way of living. The principle of such a way of living must be simple and universal. Such a principle should not be a difficult and sophisticated concept, but must be an easy and practical one which can be applied by anyone in daily life.

Mastering macrobiotic medicine means becoming a man who devotes himself in search of infinite freedom, eternal happiness, and absolute justice, and being a man who doesn't worry about money, power, knowledge, status, and fame. However skillful you are in any technique, you will be far from real freedom, happiness, and justice if your aim is money, status, or fame. This is true in the case of medicine. The more expensive the medicine becomes, the more unjust, unfree, and unhappy it becomes. Air cooled by an air-conditioner is more expensive than air in the woods, and it is harmful to us. Sunlight is cheaper and healthier than any artificial light or radiation. Water from mountain streams without pollution is much cheaper and more health-giving than soda, factory-made orange juice, or beer.

All plants grow with only sunshine, air, and water, and they are beautiful, strong and gentle. Animals are the same. The Angora rabbit of Peru has immunity to all bacterial diseases. This finding has made the animal important in medical study. It lives in the high mountains of Peru where sunlight is weak and air is thin. The secret of its immunity is that it doesn't drink much. It drinks only for necessity. Excess water makes blood thin, which in turn weakens the immune power and also thins nutrition, weakening the heart and kidneys as a result. In short, excessive and greedy eating and drinking is the cause of all sicknesses. True medicine must be cheap and can be acquired any place at any time.

Lao-tse said, "Winning without weapons is the real winning." Macrobiotic medicine is a medicine without weapons such as knives, needles, drugs, chemicals, and radiation. Macrobiotic medicine is a teaching of awareness of the reality or the Order of Nature through sickness. In this sense, macrobiotic medicine is more religious than modern religions. In fact, macrobiotic people acquire real religion, and not superstitions. In other words, when you realize that you are the cause of the sickness, and sickness is the benefactor of your life; when you like everyone, when you reach the mentality of Will Rogers who said, "I never met a man I didn't like"; when you appreciate anything including sickness, misfortune, and difficulties; then you graduate from macrobiotic medicine. To reach this state of mind, my practical method is the following:

> Live with whole grains and local, seasonal vegetables, using a bit of salt, oil, and traditional condiments.
>
> Chew each mouthful of food fifty times or more.
>
> Drink as little as possible.
>
> Work hard physically.

After three years of observing the above diet and way of living, you can firmly establish health. After that, teach macrobiotics to others for seven years. Then, devote yourself to whatever you want most in your life.

The Education of the Will

Education — East and West

Modern Western education is scientific. Its ideal is the extension of understanding through data derived from the senses — second level judgment. This education has become professional and conformist technique.

The result of modern education is apparent in the behavior of the 180 million people who populate the world. Our nation, for example, continues aerial bombardment of Vietnam fifty or sixty times a day, throws atrocious poisoned gas, uses modern chemical weapons daily that are the most murderous ever used up to the present day, and spends more than $10 million a day on this warfare.

Thus hundreds of Vietcong are killed each day. They live only on whole brown rice, and own almost no weapons. Hundreds of innocent, barefoot, wretched, pacifistic women and children die as well each day, victims of war, in this distant little country more than 10,000 kilometers from its aggressor.

In the beginning of the nineteenth century, Western education was founded on the idea that science creates superior conditions for human life. The great dream of science is that, one day, what is regarded as the greatest of all calamities — poverty — will be banished from the earth.

Far Eastern education, which originated 5,000 years ago, was completely opposite from Western education. It taught that one should enjoy poverty and consider it a blessing; that one should regard difficulties and suffering with gratitude, as a help or guide; that a simple roof sufficed for shelter and that a handful of rice and a few vegetables were sufficient as food.

It taught that one should consider cold and heat as teachers which fortify, rather than treat them as enemies; that it is not necessary to kill animals, and even less necessary to kill bacteria. It also taught that one should adapt oneself to everything and everyone, that one should treat others like a spring breeze while strengthening oneself with autumn frosts; that one should pardon others, respect others, and love everyone in the conviction that all is given inexhaustibly; that one should not hesitate to give one's life for others; that one should devote oneself to the search for truth — that is, the Unique Principle — and practice in daily life peace, purity, and respect for principles underlying macrobiotics.

Education in the Far East was profoundly spiritual, and taught that adaptation to nature is the way to arrive at Supreme Judgment. Later this was degraded by conformist and conceptual educators, who advocated a system which pretended to teach seeds and buds how to immediately become fruits and flowers. This new education produced a nationalistic robot-like people, obedient imitators, without the spirit of independence. It taught the youth of humanity to imitate the ideas and methods of the sages, which is impossible even for adults.

That's why, since the arrival of the seductive Western civilization, people immediately became slaves, not only materially but also spiritually. Thus it created a colonized people.

For the past one hundred years, Japan has accepted Western education with enthusiasm, and has put all its energy into becoming an imitator of Western civilization. This has led to the total defeat of Japan, without precedent in the history of humanity. In the schools of America, the world's biggest stronghold of Western civilization, as well as in the Japan of today, one sees an extraordinary rise of criminality, mental sickness, allergies, heart disease, cancer, iatrogenic diseases (diseases caused by medical treatment), the loss of the critical spirit, the inability to think, and the increase in retardation and uselessness in children.

Thus Far Eastern education, like that of the West, has made the Earth into a big spaceship in the form of a sphere, which flies at 10,000 km/hr carrying three billion individuals toward the depths of unhappiness, slavery, war, disease, suffering, and uncertainty. From this comes the necessity of discovering a new method of physiological and biological education.

The Fundamental Basis of All Education

At seventeen, I was struck with tuberculosis, and my condition was so serious that I was abandoned by modern medicine. I saved myself at the gates of death by the macrobiotic method, which is 5,000 years old. I would like to communicate to everyone the joy I feel that I have finally arrived at seventy-four years of age, at the end of my work, which for fifty-four years, since I was twenty years old, has been to spread this method to the entire world. This has been a self-education, as well as an education of the public.

Far Eastern medicine, originating 5,000 years ago, was not a medicine of symptoms, but a fundamental method of cure which was based on natural causes. This is why it was also a method of health, longevity, and happiness. It was not concerned with the disappearance of symptoms, but it was an educative medicine, which had as its end the development of man's judgment. This is revealed in the original theory of education of the old Chinese medicine; in the three great imperial disciplines of Japan; in the Code of Manu; in the Ayurvedic medicine of India; and in the dietary disciplines of all the great religions of humanity, such as Buddhism, Jainism, and Christianity.

The five great religions of humanity were born in the East. They are the guiding fundamental conditions, the synthesis of theory and practice, the testimonial by its own life of the unity or monism which permits the establishment of a world of peace, and the realization of the happy life that humanity desires. That is why it is quite evident that humanity must include a method of health, physiology, pathology, and medicine. But this understanding has grown dim over thousands of years, until it has been eclipsed finally and has disappeared before the importation of dualistic, materialistic, atomic, technical, modern civilization, whose judgment is based on brilliant and seductive appearances.

The primordial problem for man is the establishment of

health. This is why we must give the greatest emphasis to the education of health and hygiene. All living creatures know how to control their own health except for man. Western medicine attaches all importance to the disappearance of symptoms. It does not search for the cause, and never tries to build up the source of vitality. Consequently, it has become a simple, specialized technique; it has fallen into mere formality, and its educative spirit has completely disappeared. That is why modern medicine vegetates in an impasse, in spite of formidable technical progress. If, in days of old, one believed in this omnipotent medicine which today is represented by the American Medical Association, the dictator of America that even President Kennedy could not control, one must recognize its total defeat before these four sicknesses: cancer, heart disease, and mental and allergic conditions, which are the cause of 70 to 80 percent of all deaths in America.

But the reality is worse, for not only are the doctors incapable of curing these four great sicknesses, but they can only postpone the death of men who suffer from general sicknesses and maintain them as patients, just as they cannot cure the common cold or rheumatism, or diabetes, or eczema, or any other chronic disease. As Claude Bernard said, "The true medicine does not yet exist"; or as Bergson said, "The greatest fault of science is the ignorance of life." Dr. Rene Allendy also declared, "Pasteur, whose glory exceeds Napoleon's, has in reality weakened humanity by destroying the system of natural selection, and blemished the history of French medicine and France."

In the Far East, ancient education was, before all else, a way of independence — the study of self, physiologically and biologically — and its goal was to follow a free and peaceful way, through establishment of health by oneself, for oneself, and under one's control. The Orientals made a single way of medicine and education.

Thanks to the death of three of my nearest family members by the time I was ten years old, I vowed to discover the true cause of this absurd unhappiness, and by chance I found it. However, when I began to spread this practical method of life, I immediately encountered the second great problem of my life: the *will.*

Marx discovered that all the evils of society originated with bad distribution of food and drink; he wanted to teach the establishment of a correct system, by revolution. Scarcely sixty years after his death, this idea has become the guide of the greatest part of the world's population, yet one can see that social problems have not diminished. On the contrary, they are continuing to grow, they are taking on a horrible aspect, they have escalated to the greatest degree, and all humanity trembles in uncertainty and lives in the fear of future war.

Health, liberty, peace, and individual happiness are menaced. The hospitals and psychiatric clinics become establishments essential to city life, as temples and schools were in the past. The progress of medicine and medical paraphernalia are an indication of the increase in sickness and suffering; police reinforcement indicates the growth of criminality. This means that, although the theory of Marx has marvelously changed the structure of societies, it has forgotten the spirituality of man, the conception of the universe, and its will; that is, everything which is most essential.

If one practices macrobiotics, incurable sicknesses are eliminated and uncertainties disappear with a single blow. The four physiological and biological scourges according to Buddhism — life, sickness, old age, and death — are problems resolved. Young students amuse themselves with their studies, adults succeed in their work, all become more and more happy each day, family life is gratifying, and all life becomes more and more interesting. If one lives correctly according to macrobiotics, all will go well and world peace can be rapidly realized. But the difficulty is that most people, especially the sick, don't have the *will* to hold to such a simple macrobiotic life. They lack will to such an extent that they prefer to submit to sickness and poverty, and are driven to crime. It is therefore necessary that the spiritual education, the education of the will, precede the reconstruction of society. Even after this revolution is made, if one neglects the education of the will, one will add to the production of salaried conformists, slaves to their machines, a dependent race which passes laws for playing with the machines for all who remain passive, robot observers and live blindly. Thus, in place of the creative spirit, the spirit of imitation is substituted, because those who create themselves and their own destiny are very small in number.

The fundamental basis of education is: (1) the self-control of health, and (2) the establishment of will. The first condition is resolved by applying the macrobiotic method. But by what educative method can one fortify the will? This second condition is the great problem. What is the great secret?

What is Will?

"To want is to be able," says a French proverb.

"Clear thought leads to saintliness," says a Chinese proverb.

In all times, great men — the free men, the sages — have proclaimed the importance of the will. No one denies it; everyone agrees that this is so. Nevertheless, most of humanity fails to use the will in everyday life, and life ends tragically for man after having known only "the glory of the bindweed" (a brief, ephemeral existence).

What are the reasons for this? What is the will? Are there many kinds or levels of the will? Are there other conditions than the will alone for changing the destiny of man?

Science keeps an absolute silence on these questions. This is normal. In the conception, or rather, techniques of Western studies, the end of research is relative, limited, ephemeral, and physical. In other words, the focus is on the material world.

I posed these questions to the Far East, which has researched principally the infinite world — absolute, eternal, and constant; that is, the spiritual world. The response was the following:

1. The will is the progressive form of judgment.
2. There are seven levels of judgment, and therefore seven levels of the will:
    1. Mechanical or blind
    2. Sensorial
    3. Sentimental or emotional
    4. Intellectual
    5. Social
    6. Ideological
    7. Supreme

3. The seven steps reflect the natural development of life. For example, in a plant the development is from seed to sprout to stalk to branches to leaves to flowers to fruits. Judgment or will is vitality itself. However, the first six steps have value only in the relative, limited world. Only the seventh is valid in the absolute world, as well as the relative world.

4. Vitality, or the principle of development in nature, and the principle of the universe are the same.

5. Vitality *increases* by the mutual sympathy of the two opposing elements, yin and yang: darkness/light, humidity/dryness, dilation/compression, centrifugal force/centripetal force, etc.

6. The greatest mission of education is to make known the will, or "infinite expansion." When it is strong, it creates the man who has absolute health, who can "try without trying," "convince without speaking," "order the mountain to enter the sea," "conquer without fighting," "govern the strong with gentleness," "transmute the impossible into the possible," and "accept difficulties with joy."

Educating the Will

Since the will develops naturally and freely through seven levels, an artifical and exterior education is useless. Even though animals do not go to school, they develop in a perfect and sane way. They lead a free life, without sickness, without worries, without poverty, without scandalous pleasures. Instead of continuing the present system of education, it would be wise to discover a method of helping everyone to raise their judgment and change their thinking to one of deep appreciation and gratitude for their bosses, friends, and enemies. With this attitude it doesn't matter what we do — we are happy any time, anywhere, without the crimes and wars that men are practicing now. A small seed, which has neither force nor arms, accepts conditions of darkness, pressure, cold, and dampness. Instead of complaining or blaming others, it uses these conditions as sources of energy. It is trampled on and eaten by insects and worms, but with each difficulty it fortifies itself and develops more and more. Thus, man can lead a free life and be at peace with himself if he accepts it as a grain does;

but, on the other hand, if he looks for artificial ease, comfort, pleasure, assistance, wealth, and security, or if he has an Epicurian conception of life — in the current degraded sense of the word — he will weaken his natural vitality.

It is therefore important for education to give the opportunity and the chance to know the natural origin of health — to teach the way to achieve health in every sense of the word. This way consists of using the correct foods, combining them properly, cooking properly, and eating properly. As a consequence, one can discover and master by himself all the fundamental knowledge necessary to the social life of man, since judgment follows the process of its natural development. Those who, unhappily, have not received this education are the victims of natural selection, and will know only the suffering and difficulty of the world, the darkness of the seed and sprout. In time, many will fall in discouragement and become more and more unhappy, and manifest this unhappiness as criminals, slaves, and patients. The unhappy, the slaves, are the heavy burden of civilized society, and they can become the cause of war. The responsibility for the existence of unhappiness belongs to the low judgment of parents and educators. However, these difficulties and sufferings are the indispensable touchstone for those who have Supreme Judgment, since only these social evils can transmute discouragement into will.

Education — Past and Future

During the fifty-four years that I have devoted to macrobiotics, I have spent more than twenty of them observing the educational programs of diverse Western countries. It is evident that their education is founded on the scientific knowledge which has built their civilization. For the most part, the teachings are techniques intended to aid adaptation to life. This means that it is a *materialistic* education, adapted to the physical world.

From its origin, science has been a study of the physical world, following the research of Epicurus and Democritus. One finds systems of education founded on philosophy, religion, morals, and ideas, but these seem to be only accessories to the royal world of physics. Before the Renaissance, education was more blindly believing, mystical, and superstitious, but this approach was considered nonrealistic by the rational educational leaders who followed, and was rejected. This modern form of education is not concerned with metaphysics, and does not study spirituality, life, liberty, happiness, justice, memory, judgment, health, beauty, or art. It only treats them technically. Consequently, modern education remains impotent before the increase in vandalism and cancer, which is the cause of thirty percent of deaths among the scholar-students of Tokyo, and the appearance of twelve-year-old diabetics! Likewise, it can only impotently remain with crossed arms before wars and massacres, and likewise before the situation in America where one person in ten is struck with mental disease at least once in his life. Neither Bertrand Russell, Schweitzer, Toynbee, the Pope, Sartre, nor any politicians can find a method which stops this miserable inhuman aggression which is without parallel in history.

The leading articles in the newspapers of the "civilized" countries speak morning and night of crimes, tragedies, and accidents. But they only expose the visible part of the great iceberg of crimes, and the incapacity of modern education. The proof is that all this is never (or hardly ever) found in the countries which have not made a great profusion of this so-called education. The more civilization and education develop, the more patients, unhappiness, and atrocious professional crimes there are. Modern armaments, the biggest inventions of science, have made possible great massacres and destruction on a scale never before realized in the history of humanity. The massacres of Auschwitz and the atomic bombs of Hiroshima and Nagasaki have only been preludes. These bombs, costing $1 million each, created by the scientist Oppenheimer, have killed 314,000 persons on the battlefields of these two towns, and over the last twenty years they have slowly continued killing the survivors.

Nevertheless, Vietnam is under bombardment, which costs more than a million dollars a day! This condition of reality in Vietnam has moved and aroused the concerned Japanese youth to form the "Committee for Peace in Vietnam" which is maintained and sustained by tens of thousands of students, Buddhists, Christians, Shintoists, and even by politicians. Their action has sufficiently influenced *The New York Times* to make the appeal, "Can bombs bring peace to Vietnam?" Meanwhile, the H-bomb is capable of slaughtering 100 million persons in one explosion and can at one blow wipe from the earth whole countries like England, France, and Japan! One hundred thousand of these H-bombs are ready, of which the total capacity for destruction represents a slaughter of humanity seventy-five times over and the disappearance of all human civilization!

Contemporary world history began with the East India Company, the hunt for slaves in Africa, the landings in Goa and Hong Kong, and their occupation. The division and colonization of the countries of all races by the whites made paradise (which had been discovered by Kipling, Stevenson, and sailors who mutinied on the *Bounty*) completely disappear from the earth. That is, the "civilized" have perpetrated scenes of slaughter and destruction throughout the world, and are leading all humanity to its end, even though they believe they are capable of establishing a more beautiful and happier world. It is the clearest result of scientific civilization and the education which it founded.

It is necessary to say that there are a few rare persons among Westerners who have the capacity to self-criticize, and who have foreseen the end of humanity: Schupengrae, E. Carpenter, A. Carrell, etc. They have bewailed and prophesied the coming tragedy and the end of Western civilization and of its education, in works such as *The Failure of Western Science*, *Civilization: Its Cause and Cure*, and *Man the Unknown*.

W. Heitler, current director of the Institute of Theoretical Physics of Zurich — like Einstein, he fled Nazi Germany and took refuge in free territory — has written and published a book entitled *Man and Science*. Courageously, this wise man of modern physics insists on the necessity of forestalling humanity's demise, the biggest tragedy in history, produced by science and contemporary education.

One can make the following resume of his book. "Scientific civilization, after extraordinary progress, has resulted in spiritual insanity. To save the world from this misery un-paralleled on earth, and avert the ruin which approaches all humanity, one must before all save this science and this civilization from its stupidity and psychosis. Scientific civilization has been deluded from the start. Its research has only one end — occupation and dictatorship of the visible world, the physical world of matter, elementary particles, etc. . . . . It has forgotten that there is infinite spirituality and universal space beyond the world of limited and ephemeral particles. But what is most precious for humanity is this invisible world, the world of spirituality. Immediately, right now, we must stop all physical research and begin with all our force the dialectical research of the metaphysical world, the world of the spiritual civilization, the Order of the Infinite Universe! Here it is. The direction is given — the direction of the method which will save the contemporary generation, all humanity, all civilization, and all science."

The research of metaphysics, spirituality, will, Supreme Judgment, happiness, justice, peace, liberty, and Infinite Life was the specialty of thinkers or sages of the Far East for five thousand years. It is there that the five great religions of man were born, but these religions have since become excessively antiquated mummies. Let us lay all this aside completely and start a new edition of the world, one that is neither physical nor metaphysical, but physical *and* metaphysical *at the same time*. It must provide the simplest and most practical method, which may be understood by all immediately, and is applicable in the daily life of all races.

It is the new practical, physiological, and biological education. Its unique instrument is practical dialectics: an amusing algebra which resolves any difficult problem by employing yin and yang as the unknowns. Even children can understand it in an hour.

For fifty-four years I have studied it, I have practiced it in my daily life, I have taught it, and I have made many thousands of practitioners in all corners of the world. I have adequately confirmed this dialectic — otherwise called "the magic spectacles" — by my own practice. I have grown firm in my conviction by the confirmation that thousands of people of the scientific world, of the white race, have given me as well, after having practiced it like myself. I put the continuation of my discovery in the hands of the young people. Today, at the age of seventy-four, I am calm and free, for the first time in my life. I receive each day letters of gratitude, soaked with tears, from unknown persons, from unknown countries, from all over the world.

Education For a Peaceful World

Humanity has now ended the first chapter of its history which, from the beginning of the universe to the end of scientific civilization, comprises many thousands of years.

Its last page conforms to the prediction of the Apocalypse, in which all the predictions are realized, in order, from when the first angel sounds his trumpet to the seventh. Now is the beginning of the new world. The second chapter begins.

A new world begins with a new Genesis.

The humanity of the first Genesis tried to adapt itself to the conditions offered by nature and to create a free and peaceful life, as the animals do — fish, insects, and birds. However, man is born with a *thinking* brain, which is the difference between him and other living beings. (Why does only man have this brain which thinks? It is an important and interesting question, but I will not discuss it here.)

Because of this gift of thought, the manner of man's reply to nature's offerings takes two antagonistic forms. One is harmonious adaptation; the other is the conquest of nature.

The first begins with innocent surprise, and, passing through the mysterious, ends with the discovery of the Order of the Universe. It leads finally to the world of peace, infinite gratitude, and universal identification. The second begins with fear rather than surprise and takes the path of destruction, killing, and conquest by violence, all by way of hate.

This parallel between the faith of the Far East (the first process) and that of the West (the second) is very interesting, because both, due to low judgment which dominates everywhere, have equally and normally produced lies, illusions, fantasies, wildness, hate, and malice. An example is the division between East and West, which forms an extraordinary antagonism! Finally, the time has come for East and

West to come together. The West, whose end is conquest, came to conquer by violence the Far East, which considers adaptability as the superior way. These aggressive conquerors have run into a mutual collision of interests concerning each one's own profit at the expense of the beautiful prey which is the Far East. Thus, at present, the final scene of the miserable end of humanity is manifesting itself according to the prophecy of the Apocalypse!

But it is the time of the new beginning when all must be remade. The history of humanity is now at the first line of the first page of the second volume.

Let us re-establish a new world with our own hands. At first, re-education must be the way. This education establishes health first of all by its physiological and biological method. This is the setting in which the will appears: "a healthy spirit in a healthy body."

Peace Through Macrobiotics

The education which will produce the new world, a free and peaceful world, begins with the creation of the healthy man. It is purely physical education, the reappearance and reproduction, physically and biologically, of a total process of three billion years of evolution. After fertilization, the product of the egg and sperm increases itself three billion times in 280 days. Then the baby only grows twenty times as much in the next twenty years. Therefore, these three billion years constitute a condensed process of primordial importance in the creation of man. I believe that it would be very suitable to count this period of three billion years as the biological unit of human evolution, as a generation of life or, in other words, a "biological year."

"You are what you eat," said Francois Brillat-Savarin. From my study of Far Eastern medicine, and my fifty-four years of teaching it, I am more and more deeply and entirely convinced of the truth of these words, and I have arrived at this conclusion: *if the nourishment is just, then the man is just.*

Nevertheless, I had no way of knowing what was the correct nourishment across the unfolding march of evolution during three billion years on Earth. However, among the men who have practiced and been cured by macrobiotics with me, miracles have been produced one after another. They have had marvelous children. Even women who had never been able to have children have given birth to boys or girls according to their desire. Childbirth has been without difficulty and very rapid. The children are in perfect health, and particularly easy to raise, never catching cold. Everyone reacts with surprise when seeing them. Thus, I have discovered, without a teacher, the principle of embryology.

I know of nothing more important for a human life and for society than the nourishment of the mother during the human embryonic period. It is the time of the fundamental construction of man's life. It is the period where the three-billion-year process of evolution is condensed! I see nothing which has a greater influence on human life than this nourishment during the embryonic period. This is all that needs to be said concerning the fundamental education of man in the embryonic period.

The physiological and biological education of childhood and youth is of the greatest importance after the embryonic period. If one gives macrobiotic nourishment from this age, one will make boys and girls who fulfill the seven conditions of health. Moreover, whoever fulfills these conditions realizes, by himself and for himself, a happy life. He becomes an independent man, who studies by himself. And a woman like this will be able to establish a happy family. She will devote herself to the construction of a happy and healthy society and country. If there is one such woman in ten thousand, their country will become a country of liberty and peace. If there are but ten such countries in the world, peace on earth will be maintained forever, and one will see atrocities, mass murder, and barbarous wars (which don't exist among animals) disappear.

If all humanity desires peace — that is, a world where mass assassinations have disappeared — then there is not any other education or method more simple to realize it.

* * *

By conferences and writings everywhere in the world, I have published this educative physiological and biological method for fifty-four years. And I have obtained more than sufficient confirmation of its efficacy; the examples of it are many. They have been published in old reviews and books. Here are a few of them:

1. Mr. William Dufty, a fifty-year-old American, holder of the highest honors from England, France, and Switzerland, former officer of aviation, hospitalized for more than ten years after the second World War, who no longer knew what to do with his body which was like a living corpse, weighed 80 kilograms (176 pounds). He began to practice macrobiotics two years ago by following the directions in my books. He lost 37 kilos in six months and looks twenty years younger. In gratitude he has decided to devote his life to macrobiotics. He has translated and published *You Are All Sanpaku*, which required one year of work, but it has earned him a good reputation. He has declared that he will translate all of my works in order to present them to the West.

2. Miss Cuilitz of Brussels, after having found a new conception of life through macrobiotics, has offered me a villa and apartments which are worth 20 million yen ($80,000).

3. An American girl, Miss Pletersky of New York, saved by macrobiotics from a miserable death, saved for two years the money necessary for a pilgrimage to Japan, but she offered this money to Vietnamese macrobiotics. This is a living example of the transmutation of the conception of life.

4. Mrs. Teal Ames, an American actress, quit her work to devote all her fortune and herself to the establishment of a macrobiotic food distribution center, Chico-San Incorporated, in America. In this center, she worked on the production of a whole grain macrobiotic bread, exactly like Cinderella (so well that a prince appeared and took her away in his pumpkin coach!).

5. Mrs. Simon, twenty-four years old, a young American artist, innocent as an angel or a child, was one among hundreds of thousands of Americans who threw themselves too fanatically into macrobiotics. The beautiful letters that she wrote me for the first time, just before her death, teach us vividly of her character.

At the beginning of February 1965, she began macrobiotics with her husband, and in nine weeks they were miraculously saved from terrible incurable sicknesses, caused by bad eating and drugs they had been using for ten years. Mrs. Simon had neurosis, allergy, and heart disease; her husband had depression, tuberculosis, hardening of the arteries, and narcosis. While following macrobiotics, they added various other diets as well. She died in October! It is well known in the East that often this type of woman-child, innocent and pure as a white pearl, lacks self-reflection and ends her life tragically. Her father was president of the lawyers' association. He was against the "macrobiotics of the Rising Sun" and triggered off a massive campaign in the press, the magazines and the radio. The sale of my books was forbidden and the macrobiotic movement condemned. Mr. Dufty, as the editor of *You Are All Sanpaku*, was also accused, as well as Mrs. Irma Paule, the secretary-general of the Ohsawa Institute. This was an undoubted advance for the movement in America. Because of this event, macrobiotics in America has increased.

Mrs. Simon was an innocent, faithful, and well-loved woman. But with her simplicity and honesty, she lacked judgment and deep thought. Fatally, she came to this tragic end because she had no comprehension of the theory, although she was so enthusiastic about the practice.

Her case shows that *philosophy without technique is useless and technique without philosophy is dangerous.*

When one introduces a new idea or theory, the danger of accidents of this kind is inevitable. Theory without practice, philosophy without technique are useless. Technique and science without theory or philosophy are dangerous. It is the same with medicine, education, politics, industry, and agriculture if there is no principle — which means the First Principle: the Great Justice, the Principle of Life (health, beauty, happiness, liberty, justice); in other words, the Order of the Infinite Universe. It is unbelievable but true that modern medicine ignores life! Politics has no other end than the monopoly of rights, profit-making, and the use of violence. Industry, commerce, and agriculture are deluded in considering profit as primary. It is especially unpardonable that agriculture, whose purpose is the production of the sustenance of life, has profit as an end, and the unceasing increase in financial returns. The first constitution of Japan states formally that agriculture is the base of politics, and one of the three sacred rules in the formation of Japan established the National Order of Agriculture according to macrobiotic living.

The Unique State
Called Happiness

What pleasure you seem to derive from drowning yourselves in the pool of sensory judgment! But do not fret — you are not alone. Even the President of the United States, the leaders of Soviet Russia, Bertrand Russell, and Gandhi have made extraordinary strides in the same realm. Be grateful that until now you have not been made the victims of blind judgment, like the seven million human sacrifices of the last war.

From the age of twenty, I have not ceased to follow the narrow path. I am in a state of soul that is extremely calm and joyous. Seventh Heaven, the universe of infinite development cannot elude us — it is no longer out of reach. Courageous men and women! Be strong! Step by step you can travel the unique way to the very summit.

Achieving Happiness

There are many methods for achieving a happy life. Many of them come from the Orient and are spiritual. They run the gamut from ascetic religious training to the physical gymnastics of Yoga. There are hygenic and medical methods such as Occidental science, yet there are few that have happiness as their final goal.

A Swiss scholar named Hilty has called his approach *Happiness*. It is motivated, however, by spiritual, moral, Christian culture that is difficult to apply consistently for most people.

Methods like Marxism that promise the establishment of happiness in our material lives through social revolution or violent action are offering false hope. Many people know this already. The others will understand sooner or later.

We still have not found the scientific means to achieve happiness. On the contrary, what is called the *happy life* absolutely cannot come into being by way of science. The end of scientific civilization and the destruction of all of humanity *can* be the end result of thermonuclear war.

Nonetheless, you know that I do not make light of either social or scientific revolution. Many of you can vouch for the fact that I am likely to be in the forefront of either one. I openly declare that I am a man who does not oppose social revolution, civilization, or development in science. I have great respect for even an invention like the atomic bomb, and I admire grandiose thermonuclear warfare.

I for one applaud both creativity and destruction. I would never hesitate to support any effort, however misdirected, if its goal were infinite liberty and eternal happiness.

I would not hesitate to offer all my admiration to even the medical conformist who earns his living by consuming the very life-blood of the most pitiable people on earth — ignorant slaves. Conversely, I proffer my sympathy and pity to those conformists upon such science and medicine.

Yet I am content not to have played the game of these politicians, doctors, and revolutionists. To tell the truth, I was born a tragic character destined to end in tragedy at the head of a catastrophically sensational revolutionary movement. I inherited this character from my mother, who died very young.

She passed away after having totally and gallantly followed a way of life based on the new science. I firmly maintain this spirit of my mother even now.

I believe that all men live with the spirit of their mothers as their principal driving force. The influence of the father is much less important. Twenty years ago I wrote a long poem as a eulogy to my mother. I live in the spirit of that poem even today. For seventy years, all my words and achievements have been merely the actualization of that maternal essence.

In short, *this has been the behavior of one who hungers and thirsts for Justice.* I live from morning to night (at night in my dreams) without being separated from my mother for an instant. I have lived at each instant for the realization of my mother's aims; this will continue to the end of my life.

My mother had lived her poor life believing with all her heart that scientific civilization, medicine and modern hygiene were in actuality Justice. All Japanese, for that matter, believe that Occidental science teaches Justice and the essentials of life (the very things they have come to take for granted in the traditional philosophy of the Orient). In reality, Occidental methods are only techniques.

In traditional China, happiness is thought to depend on five conditions:

1. Longevity — a long life
2. Detachment from money — not to be overly influenced by wealth
3. Security
4. Cultivation of one's character and virtue
5. Thinking unceasingly of ways to achieve the greatest and most marvelous thing, e.g.,
   a. re-establishing the health of one's body
   b. re-establishing order in one's family
   c. establishing a peaceful government
   d. guiding the whole world towards Justice.

Occidental happiness is quite another thing. Webster's large dictionary as well as the Larousse and the Littre Encyclopedia discuss happiness at length and reach these surprising conclusions: that happiness can never be achieved in this world, that it is a matter of luck, that perfect happiness does not exist on this earth, etc., etc.

My conclusion about Occidental definitions of happiness is:

1. Wealth
2. Wealth
3. Wealth
4. Wealth
5. Wealth

In short, money is happiness. Gold, silver, fortune, the treasures that Christ scorned have become the most important, precious things in the world. Thus, it is natural that science has become the most important study, that industry is most powerfully active. It is also natural that they could lead humanity into total war. In other words, intellectual judgment has replaced Supreme Judgment at the head of the list in the Occident.

I do not imply that intellectual judgment (the fourth level) is evil. If the Occident, however, were to reach social, then ideological, and lastly Supreme all-encompassing Judgment, science itself might produce even more miracles.[11]

The Orient, which teaches Supreme Judgment from the very outset (considering the other six to be of little importance), has been totally colonized by Occidental civilization, as we can plainly see.

In Japan, however, sentimentality (the third level of judgment) is remarkably well developed. In matters of love, the guiding principle is the law of Supreme Judgment: all or nothing. Even in popular songs it is evident: "Fear not, I am yours even if it means plumbing the lowest depths of hell."

Paul Claudel, former French consul in the Orient, has left an extraordinary collection of traditional popular songs of this type.

Love in the modern world is either at the first (blind) level of judgment like that of amphibious plankton, or at the second (sensory) level like that of cats or dogs: it is no more than superficial, spontaneous, sexual.

If one does not have the emotional strength to live through this blind and sensory love, one cannot come to that of the sentimental (third) or intellectual (fourth) level.

To love is to make one's mate happy. The happiness of which I speak is really infinite liberty, absolute justice, eternal joy. This implies loving *all* — humanity, animals, vegetables. It is the universal love described by Erasmus — love at the highest (seventh) level.

If you have not tasted the joy of loving *one* person with all your heart, with all your might, you cannot imagine the infinite joy of the love of which Erasmus speaks — universal love or sadness. To understand, one has to have experienced the unbearable sorrow of being betrayed by his loved one.

In the spring, one falls in love — the miraculous product of the yin-yang polarization of the Sixth Heaven. This should blossom into unlimited, infinite, absolute love. Unfortunately, we arrest this development and concretize it at the blind or sensory level.

If you want to know the true character of judgment of a man, observe his behavior in love.

* * *

The condition that for me is the great, unique, characteristic of happiness is not that of the Chinese definition, nor that of the Swiss, Hilty, of Descartes, Schopenhauer, or even Erasmus. Summed up, it is *to be human.*

It is the establishment of free will. To be human signifies that one has mastered the logarithmic spiral of the Order of the Universe, to which I have consecrated my whole life.

The different aspects of this world are due to the differentiation of the One aspect of the Infinite or absolute. The origin of man is universal soul or spirit, the functions of which are memory, judgment, and will.

The six levels that manifest themselves between the nondifferentiated world and the relative, differentiated world are the path or way of the eternal, logarithmic spiral in which man must accomplish a voyage in and out.

In other words, the true happiness of man is to explore precisely his native land — Seventh Heaven or Infinity. It is to clearly know the meaning of Oneness, to experience the fact that the soul is One, that all things in this world are indivisible despite the fact that human beings are apparently separate from one another, and made up of billions and billions of cells. Here is the meaning of Unity, the concept of the identity of all humanity, the unification of the entire world.

Having arrived at that point, one cannot distinguish others, and from then on, there is no separation. In the whole world all are reunited in *One;* the term *others* no longer exists. There is neither strife, jealousy, rancor nor envy. Therefore, if someone experiences the sentiment of compassion or mercy towards *others*, he is an exclusive dualist!

The Macrobiotic Bond

Those who breathe the same oxygen, who warm themselves at the same fire, who drink from the same source, who live and nourish themselves on the milk and blood of the same earth, who are born of the same womb, are brothers and sisters. This brother and sister relationship, not a product of law or violence to begin with, cannot be broken by law or violence. Even more strongly so, the relationship between parents and children, between compatriots, between man and wife, between master and disciple, between intimate friends, cannot be broken during the length of one's life. Even if there is a clash of opinions or ideas, at the very most it is a contradiction peculiar to the first six levels of judgment. On the seventh level, there is no opposition and no need for separation.

In the realm of seventh judgment, there is no possession, no separation, no despair, no promises, no duties, no rights. It is a world without contracts, the world of freedom, the world of the identity of self and others — the soul of millions of individuals. He who speaks in terms of opposition and separation is an opportunist and a dualist. He attests to his ignorance of the absolute and of Infinity.

Macrobiotic friends throughout the world; friends who walk together on the road to infinite liberty, eternal happiness, and absolute justice, who are joined by a stroke of fortune that is extremely rare in this world; *do not separate. Do not abandon one another.* There is no reason to discard a friend even if his comprehension is of the lowest sort, because infinite liberty, absolute justice and eternal happiness are *One.* There lies the realm of monism. If you abandon your friends, family or teacher, it indicates that you are venturing into the world of opposition, the world of low judgment and dualism. Never separate, even if you are in conflict and struggling terribly with one another.

A brother is always a brother even after death. If you find shortcomings in your friends, you can help them to change by seeking the cause of the problem. If you cannot make them see the light, your judgment has not yet reached the seventh level. You must redouble your efforts to improve *yourself.*

Gratitude is always gratitude — even for a glass of water or a bowl of rice. A debt of gratitude must be repaid ten thousand times over or it will weigh you down forever. You are ungrateful, arrogant, exclusive. Master Ishizuka [Ohsawa's teacher of macrobiotic medicine] rescued me from a mortal illness. Consequently, I dedicated my life to saving ten million existences as a testimony of my gratitude: "One grain, ten thousand grains." For me, ten thousand people represent the world. *One grain, ten thousand grains* is not, in reality, the mere discharge of a debt of gratitude. It is the realization of one's Self in happiness, liberty, and justice. Only those individuals who follow this way can become citizens of the land of infinite liberty, eternal happiness, absolute justice.

* * *

These reflections on the unique state of happiness are lengthier than I had wished; I am so clumsy in expressing myself. Furthermore, it is sad that the unique state of happiness should of necessity have to be described in a negative, passive way, with phrases that begin with "it is not necessary. . ."

The path of macrobiotics and the Unique Principle, to which I have consecrated my life, is not a discipline that requires admonishments like "Thou shalt not," in the manner of Moses' Ten Commandments. My path is without condition or limit. I have made a point of not using imperatives. The only condition or obligation or discipline that is more or less mandatory in macrobiotic practice is *chew thoroughly!*

Nevertheless, just as in a moral discipline, I tell you, "Do not abandon one another, there is no need to give up." Obviously, this is a recommendation that is absolutely unnecessary for people with Supreme Judgment.

This condition is actually useless in any case; there is no choice but to allow those people to leave who must. The ones who abandon our monistic, unique path are dualists; inhabitants of the plankton and animal worlds. Slowly, one after the other, they struggle upward toward Seventh Heaven after having wasted several hundred million years. It is absolutely useless to advise them to imitate those with higher judgment. It is absurd and unhelpful. Such advice can be useful only to those who are near Seventh Heaven, who single it out like a beacon in the dark night.

To suffer from doubts as to the efficacy of macrobiotics is the normal punishment for those who have not practiced it seriously for ten years. *One deviation erases the effectiveness of the preceding practice.*

A man of low judgment often concludes that the macrobiotic dialectic of the Unique Principle (the crystallization of Supreme Judgment) is a childish, simplistic concept. To him it is suspect since it is not open to precise experimental study. This kind of opinion is precisely a reflection of simplistic, infantile arrogance.

Nuclear physics, at the conclusion of precise experimental study, has reached the conclusion that the fundamental unity of the universe is formed out of protons, neutrons, electrons, etc. This is nothing but dualism or pluralism. And here we stand at the brink of mass suicide!

Here lies buried the tale of a long voyage on the road called Low Judgment. Science suspects this. We can only hope that it will soon find its way to monism.

The Way of Life

As you see, macrobiotic cures are very simple, but sicknesses are very complicated. None of them can be cured with one treatment or operation. They have many symptoms, may change form or location, and even evolve into other sicknesses. Some people say that bacteria and viruses are the only cause of disease. This belief is based on ignorance and superstition. Even total destruction of dysentery, tuberculosis, or syphilis bacteria, say, does nothing to change the patient's vulnerability to these or other diseases. It is impossible to live joyfully and happily at the expense of destroying some other so-called harmful form of life.

Other people emphasize heredity. This is either an excuse, or an unwitting confession of incapable doctors, or a cover-up for ignorance.

Furthermore, the act of destruction is cruel and violent. It reveals dualistic thinking. Destroying living beings as a means to a peaceful life is a logical absurdity. If you see all life as one, whole and integral, then you understand that destruction is a self-centered, schizophrenic exploitation. Creation is not a self-defeating, perverted process that leads man or other animals to mass slaughter.

A lion devouring a hare is first of all a rare occasion and one that teaches the hare to understand instinctually the way of this world. Note that the hare was becoming extinct for quite some time just because he did not know how to defend himself. And the "lower" animals never wage all-out wars on each other. Enough preaching about the superiority of man. The essential thing is the simplicity of following this oldest way of eating to heal any sickness without resorting to brutal destruction. This way of eating means understanding the biological and physiological basis of a happy and healthy existence. Study this basic concept seriously and carefully.

In both theory and practice, training in macrobiotic medicine with the aid of this book appears very simple. Actually, this oldest and most dynamic philosophy is quite inaccessible to the professionally-educated Western mind. Absolute cure, I believe, comes not with the disappearance of symptoms but with the understanding of Vedantic life and the Unifying Principle. By following sattvic eating, your life becomes an example of Krishna's teaching, as it is shown in the *Bhagavad-Gita.*

The way of eating is like raja yoga when it leads us to heal others. The only way to become human — healthy, happy, and free — is by helping others heal themselves, follow the way of eating and become healthy, happy, free men and women. Only then is your life a revelation of infinite freedom, eternal happiness, and absolute integrity. You will feel infinite love for all people and you will be happy anywhere, any time.

If you are a truly free man, all others should admire you, love you, and follow your ways, including your eating.

With the compass of yin and yang, you will find the just solution in harmony with the situation. There is no need for me to elaborate; necessity is the mother of invention. Without this compass we rob and kill ourselves and each other.

You have discovered the compass, the *Weltanschauung* (universal wisdom). Assimilate it and master it so you can use it to cure any sickness and unhappiness. Your cup will flow over!

Giving

To eat is to live. To live is to give.

Remember the Order of the Universe: we of the animal world were born of the vegetal. Animals are converted vegetables, hemoglobin being a transmutation of chlorophyll. Just as plants take their sustenance from the world of elements above them, so we in the animal world below feed upon and are nourished by the multitude of plant life.

What do we give? All things exist for the purpose of giving life to higher beings. Just as the elements give freely to bring forth the vegetal, and plants proliferate and give themselves to form the animal, so we of the animal world must follow their sublime example, in utmost harmony with the Order of the Universe.

We must give. Give freely. Give everything. Give all, with pleasure in the giving. To give that of which you are possessed of plenty is not a true gift. To give truly means to deprive yourself of something dear and necessary.

Accepting

Accept everything. Illness is a blessing, a guarantee of order. Without order there could be no disorder. Accept your illness with gratitude.

Accept misfortune as you do a bonanza, knowing that it befell you because of some need or lack in you. Be grateful if your error or omission is pointed out, brought home to you. Accept war as you do peace, accept poverty like prosperity, foe like friend. He who embraces an enemy is the freest of all men.

The Western Ideal

"You must change your life," wrote Rilke in "Archaic Torso of Apollo."

You must change your life. Such was the import of an archaic fragment of the Greek ideal upon a modern poet. Apollonian perfection once, but headless now, and without arms or legs.

"It is best not to be born," the sages sang, on the crest of a Golden Age. And little wonder. Athenian intellect grafted reason and logic upon the natural tree of man, and a material philosophy flowered; the Western world is its fruit. The towers of Illium crumbled; Greek civilization declined; the glory that was Rome could not temper the barbarian's sword. The elixir of life is not found in rationality.

Heraclitus spoke out, but his message was unheeded:

> The way up and the way down is one and the same, and wisdom is learning that all things are one. God is day and night, winter and summer, war and peace, surfeit and hunger; and He takes various shapes, just as fire, when it is mingled with spices, is named according to the savor of each.

What is at variance agrees with itself. It is the opposite which is good for us. Cold things become warm, and what is warm cools; what is wet dries, and the parched is moistened. It scatters and it gathers; it advances and retires.

The twentieth century is materialism's legitimate heir. The Hellenic tradition in the West obtains today, despite the continuing lessons of two millennia — strife, warfare, bloodshed.

Reason and logic are yet enthroned, but, in truth, over whom do they rule? What is their domain, and where are their subjects? Where can one single subject be found? Better the old pantheon of capricious gods meddling in the affairs of men than materialism's gross, life-denying aims. Industrialization, science, technocracy, and progress are some of the new gods' names, and each bears its own built-in mechanical Vulcan for forging mankind's glittering new chains.

Freedom

Detach yourself from anything and everything not actually necessary for your bare existence. *Vivere parvo.* Do not depend upon anything or anybody. Depend upon yourself alone. So long as you carry a tin of aspirin in your pocket you are not free. Aspirin is no cure, only a palliative. Each five grains of aspirin you take destroys a million brain cells. Take no drugs of any kind.

A headache is the first signal of a yin imbalance in your body's chemistry. Aspirin, another yin, increases the disorder. Yangize yourself, instead. Stop drinking for a day. The headache will disappear and your system will welcome the return of its natural balance.

Macrobiotic Consciousness

All doors are closed to you. There is no place to hide. The solution is simple: become macrobiotic.

William Blake said, "If the doors of perception were cleansed, everything would appear infinite." Be macrobiotic. The essences of all things shine and sing; edges are sharp and defined yet all is one. The quantity and quality of life are enhanced, a unique awareness comes. The senses receive truly.

How pure and perfect is the smallest thing, and its counterpart; the yin and the yang — magnificent! The liberty of imagination and impulse, the depth and breadth of reality, the infinite, once glimpsed are never forgotten.

Half-beings become whole. One foot is forever in the Infinite.

See with the brightening glance, know the dancer from the dance.

Impressions are clear, clean, precise and joyous; the senses receive and transmit freely; the memory is liberated. The ruts of old thought patterns are erased and direct action follows without jolt or interference. Whatever you desire is yours. But note that your desires have changed.

All is clear. Clarification of reality is man's freedom. Absolute truth, absolute justice reigns, and no falsity exists. You will judge for yourself everything forever after. No law, causal or man-made, will command your adherence until you test it in the light of your changed self. Old truths are re-examined and discarded if false; the new truth is infinite.

When the doors of perception are cleansed, reality is sharp and clear and perfect. Color is infinite; all things radiate it. Man's history lies plain upon his face. There are no secrets. Light and dark are interchangeable, are one; the cosmos is in flux, expanding and receding tides of air.

Be macrobiotic!

The Secret of Macrobiotic Medicine

Mr. Chitarangia is sixty-three years old. He is one of the revolutionaries of India. He was jailed several times. He has a strong will. He practiced a pure vegetarian diet (nothing but vegetables, fruits, and water) for twenty-three years in order to improve his health and mentality.

After studying macrobiotics with me, two hours every day for ten months, he changed the diet to the macrobiotic diet. He is observing a strict macrobiotic diet now, which consists of ten ounces of millet, less than five ounces of vegetables, salt, and sesame oil. He doesn't urinate more than twice a day. It is I who worry about his too-strict observation of the diet. One night, Lima did palm diagnosis on his shoulder while I was talking with him.

He said, with uneasy attitude, "Why do you put your palm on my shoulder? If it is for healing, please stop it."

Lima answered, "No, I am checking where the sickness is and how your sickness is improving."

After that he was contented. He didn't want any symptomatic cure because he knows his sickness is the punishment of the Order of the Universe. His attitude is the secret of macrobiotic medicine.

There is no real cure except self-reflection and the realization that sickness is one's own fault. Punishment for the fault must be accepted even though such punishment may seem unjust. No excuses. Even when you are resented, envied, or scolded by mistake or misunderstanding, you should not make any excuses because there is no excuse in nature. *Only man makes excuses.* There is no need to excuse the Order of the Universe because it is perfect and makes no mistakes. Justice reveals itself.

One who excuses does not understand the Order of the Universe at all. Man was born in the world of freedom, love, and peace, where the Order of the Universe is called Justice. We are living without awareness of the Order. This Order can neither be disturbed nor distorted. Millions of tons of bombs may destroy all the towns on earth, and make the sky dirty for awhile. However, nature will clean up the sky again.

Man creates dirt, poisons, and unhappiness. Man exhales poisonous gas sixteen times every minute. He secretes two to three pounds of stinky liquid and waste every day. Some men are brave enough to cause war, sickness, and social violence. Most of them consume thirty million pounds of matter during their lifetime. The destruction of man is huge and enormous. However, it is allowed.

God made man to be destructive and create unhappiness. However, God also made man to be aware and observe infinite freedom, eternal happiness, and absolute justice. Man's destruction is limited and infinitesimally small compared with the greatness of the Wholeness — God. Man's work is to join God's creation. Other things, such as making money, business, fighting, sickness, etc., are only things to lead man to unhappiness. Once you understand the exactness and justness of the infinite universe and smallness of man, you will not dare to excuse any of your own faults.

Mr. Doger, the younger brother of Mr. Chitarangia, was jailed because he marched at the head of the protesting demonstration against killing cows. He was in jail for over 100 days without any court action. With his status and money it would have been easy for him to be released. However, he is a man of no excuse. He stayed in an uncomfortable jail without any complaints or excuses, while giving me permission to stay in his marbled mansion and to use his luxurious car. Furthermore, he was helping me to get status so that I could stay in India permanently.

Many famous people came to see him every day in jail to salute him. However, he didn't ask anybody to get him out of jail. He is a man of no excuse.

These two brothers know the Order of the Universe which has absolute justice. They have complete faith in the Order. This faith and the attitude of "no excuse" are the secret of macrobiotic medicine.

Your Biography Before Birth

Life Before Birth

When were you born? What year? What month? What day? Where were you 300 days before your birth? What did you look like? Where were you thirty years before your birth? When will you die?

Who knows?

You will die in twenty-four hours!

Improbable . . .

Yes, in twenty-four hours you will die. In one hour, two hours, five or six hours, in any event, in twenty-four hours, definitely. But what I would like to know is, where will you be three years after your death?

The earth will have reclaimed me.

Then you say that you have come from the earth?

No, I have come from my parents.

Then where did Man come from?

We do not know.

Where did you come from, Man, and where are you going? Where were you, what did you look like, what did you think, what did you do 300 days, 365 days, two years, three years or thirty years before your birth? And 300, 3,000, or 30,000 years before, where were you? Nowhere? We cannot answer in this way since down deep we sense that Man was *somewhere*. And we feel that we will be *somewhere* in a year, two years, five years, forty-nine years. Now and then, one involuntarily lets slip, "I will be reborn seven times . . ."

Why do we say "seven times?" Why not "eight times," "eighty

times," or "800 times?" It is because the number seven signifies non-fulfillment, eternal non-fulfillment. In the Orient, "eight" often signifies "realization." The motto "eight volumes" is an example. Also, the motto "seven and one-half volumes." (There is the story of the samurai Tawara-Tota. With a single arrow, he slew a great monster that had entwined itself around Mount Oomi-Fuji seven times.)

Nevertheless, I know that Man is reborn seven times and these seven times repeat themselves seventy times and these repeat themselves 700 times. Jesus knew it. "I will forgive you even if you sin seven times — God will forgive you even if you sin seventy times seven."

True rebirth is the rebirth of Man; it is the rebirth of the spirit or of an idea. If the spirit is not reborn, it is not a real rebirth. If the spirit is reborn, the body is partially reborn and the appearance changes. Everyone knows it instinctively.

The saying goes, "It is impossible for you to do anything without being reborn."

But the rebirth that one sees is that of the body. We sense that rebirth of the body is difficult, whereas rebirth of the spirit is easy. We often say, "By changing my spirit, I might be . . ."

Our body and spirit are reborn each day. Every day we eat fruits, leaves, roots, vegetables and grasses. These plants, along with oxygen and water, change into what we know as the human body. We couldn't live without them. Plants die, decompose in our bodies and are miraculously reborn as the human being.

Plants themselves are the outgrowth of the various earth atoms that have finished their atom-life. The atoms, in turn, are the rebirth of the elements. The elements come from energy just as energy is the product of bi-polarity.

Then what is reborn from Man?

Always Zen-nin, "the Virtuous Self," Man — more and more virtuous, more and more free, more and more righteous, more and more happy. That is why Man, as long as he has not become perfect, absolutely virtuous, infinitely free and eternally happy, looks for the path of rebirth. In reality, every man wants to be reborn, the sooner the better.

The objective of Man's rebirth is freedom and happiness.

Each night's sleep is the return to his point of departure on the voyage of rebirth. If he does not prepare himself adequately during sleep, he will fail. Conversely, with good preparation, time and space present no difficulty.

* * *

The 300th day before Man's birth is the last point of departure from the other world to this one. He who has not understood the secret of the trip cannot discover the technique of rebirth.

We are going to make a study of that 300 days before birth, the starting point of life, by means of a text written by Margaret Shea Gilbert, *The Biography of the Unborn* (Hafner, New York, 1962).

By examining in detail the growth process of Man in his mother's womb, we can know with precision what occurs behind the mystic curtain that covers the true aspect of life.

To that end, let us study embryology with the Unifying Principle — yin and yang. In so doing, we acknowledge, on the one hand, the value of the analytical, microscopic technique of embryology, medicine, physiology and anatomy as developed in the Occident. On the other, we discover the special value of the philosophy of the Far East, the principle of a free, peaceful, wholesome and happy life. It is a technique for living one's daily life which was developed in the Orient over a period of some thousands of years.

Surprisingly, this valuable tool has not been fully exploited in the realm of physiology and anatomy. Until now, it has not been applied to the study of the embryo.

Life in the Womb

The story begins with the egg (ovum) and the sperm.

From the day that she begins menstruating, a female produces one egg per month — 400 to 500 eggs during her entire lifetime (until her menstruation ends at the age of forty-nine). If we could mature all of these eggs in an incubator, one woman could be mother to 500 babies!

Since the human female is pregnant for nine months, however, she can only bear thirty-five babies during her life, hypothetically speaking.

By contrast, the male emits several hundred million sperm at a time and is capable of this massive production beyond the age of sixty.

If we sterilized all men and preserved the sperm of only one male, all the women in the world could be certain of being impregnated.

It is common knowledge that often only a single bull is put into a pasture because bulls are greedy and violent and are not as useful, economically, as cows or steers. In fact, at times we dispense with the bull entirely and resort to artificial insemination. If we were to apply this method to man, who in his greed and violence closely resembles the bull, war and murder would decrease without a doubt!

In the realm of fish, the female produces several million eggs, most of which are eaten or destroyed. Since, however, quantity favors the species, whether among men or fish, it would seem that nature anticipated this situation.

In a typical human ovum, almost fully developed, the tiny cells at the periphery are the nutrition cells. The shape of the ovum is round (yang); that of the sperm is elongated (yin). The fact that the ovum descends and the sperm ascends makes the former yang and the latter yin. According to the Unifying Principle, it is evident that the yang ovum comes from the yin female and the yin sperm from the yang male. Yin produces yang and yang produces yin.

The yin female attracts yang; then she ejects that which is yang, after having utilized it to the utmost, because her nature is originally yin. The ovum and sperm are the evacuations of nature.

The egg ripens and descends once a month. If it makes contact with the sperm in the Fallopian tube, it arrives in the womb at the end of about three days. Conception begins.

Embryology ignores the following questions:

1. How do the egg and sperm meet?
2. Why does the sperm travel ten centimeters in one hour while the egg takes three days to cover the same distance?
3. Why is it that, under normal circumstances, only a single sperm out of billions will penetrate the egg?

These unresolved problems are very exciting if studied in the light of the Unifying Principle.

By the end of the first month, the egg becomes fifty times larger and weighs 8,000 times more than it did at the start.

The day they unite, the egg and sperm form a single cell. At the end of a month, an organism has been formed that is six millimeters in length, with a head, a thorax, a tail and all the organs necessary for life. The fertilized egg doubles and redoubles; it multiplies dozens of millions of times.

All animals reproduce by division and this phenomenon is endless. Dr. Alexis Carrel was awarded the Nobel prize for his studies of the heart of an embryo chicken. He found that the heart continued its development indefinitely if one preserved it in a special environment.

The power of division is astonishing. When it has been arrested, death occurs. The force of division is brought to a standstill by its opposition — contraction and immobilization.

In actuality, the cell world is dialectic. It is an uncertain world where these opposite forces interact. This is the fundamental mechanism of life.

Sensation, emotion, thought and judgment also depend on this interaction. Consequently, we can say that all existence is dialectic: cold-warm, joy-anger, love-hatred, pleasure-discomfort, peace-war, material-spiritual, good-bad, liberty-slavery, good fortune-adversity, right-wrong. It is useless to seek the absolute (peace, justice, liberty, and happiness) in the relative world since the absolute can be neither limited nor uncertain.

Man, in general, was not able to unlock this secret during the three billion physiological years spent in his mother's womb.

In the Orient long ago, the few who were able to discover this secret did not teach it to everyone. And they were right. It is something that cannot be taught precisely. It can only be grasped when one has discovered oneself.

Strangely enough, when an attempt was made to teach it, no one understood! And yet, everyone instinctively knows the absolute, the Infinite. Unfortunately, we seek without comprehension because our judgment is veiled.

* * *

The first cell continues its division indefinitely, but it changes its direction and its manner of progression according to circumstances, and it stops on its own at a naturally determined limit.

Man grows three to five billion times during the 280 days of gestation. He comes into the world when division can go on no longer in the environment of the womb.

After birth, he grows only twenty times more. His total growth is more than 60 to 100 billion times the size of the first cell. This is the final growing point of the relative world. From that time on, if there is a part of the body that continues to grow or divide, that growth or division is abnormal — the malady called cancer. Under other circumstances, this unnatural division manifests itself in tragic behavior: arrogance, greed, treachery.

Mental illnesses are the result of this sort of body malfunction.

However, if the divisive, centrifugal force of the first cell is channeled in a spiritual direction, it moves freely toward the absolute and eternal world and settles in Supreme Judgment.

The two forces which between them produce cancer, stop cell division and determine the direction which growth follows, are called yin and yang. Yin is the divisive force while yang is the contractive force that moderates and changes direction.

Anyone can control left or right, contraction or expansion, if he deeply understands the workings of these two forces. Centrifugal and centripetal force are the causes of our birth into the relative world. In the body, in diet, in existence, these forces take various forms. We can make what we want of our lives by controlling them.

One can interpret this truth as either mystical idealism or categorical materialism since it appears that we blend the material and spiritual world. That is why our starting point is embryology.

Diet and Fetal Development

Diet is the most important factor in the phenomena of life and physiology and especially in the phenomena of life and physiology in the womb of the mother. Its importance is inestimable. In the development of the fetus we clearly see the influence of yin and yang, expansion and contraction. The proportions of these two factors in food determine the shape of all creation.

Salt, for example, is very yang. It toughens and brings things together. It can be used anywhere, at any time. If one cooks beans with a little salt, it is difficult to soften them. If one adds some salt before cooking potatoes, they do not lose their shape.

Many elements are antagonistic to the forces of salt — for example, water, sugar, potassium, sulphur, oxygen, and nitrogen. If potatoes are cooked with much water or some sugar, they become a shapeless mass.

Today, radishes, sweet potatoes, rice and wheat are larger (more swollen) than in former years because they are cultivated with chemical fertilizers (sulfur, nitrogen, phosphorus, water) — all antagonistic to salt.

Yet, without the elements that soften, disjoin and separate them, vegetables and man become small, rigid and dwarflike instead of growing abundantly. They are similar to radish miso-zuke (vegetables preserved in miso or salt under pressure for two or three years) or dried codfish.

In the plastic arts, we call the balance of yin and yang the Golden Proportion, that which creates the most esthetic form.

In physiology, the Golden Proportion is seven parts yin to one part yang. A body that has this balance is a sound one.

The Child With a Hare-Lip

To demonstrate the effects of yin and yang on the fetus, let us look at the case of a child born with a hare-lip. Official medicine can offer no explanation or cure for this tragic affliction. Yet by the Unique Principle of yin and yang it can be understood.

Everyone comes into the world with a hare-lip. Ordinarily, the right and left halves of the upper lip are drawn to one another, joining in the middle. The lip channel under the nose is the vestigial remains of this split, the channel marking the line of juncture.

During the first month of gestation, every embryo has a hare-lip. At the end of the second month, it is gone. If, during that period, the prospective mother does not eat foods that give the lip parts the power to unite, or if she eats anything that weakens that power, her baby will have a hare-lip. This is independent of the quantity of food she takes.

Even if the juncture occurs, it can easily be undone, since at first it is soft and delicate. It can be undone if the mother eats foods that upset the process that is going on.

Food that produces hare-lip is that which contains 10 or 70 times more yin elements than yang ones. Evidently, it is not a problem that involves one single food but a general problem of yin-yang balance in all foods. Calculating for every food is very complicated. It is not so difficult, however, to figure the proportion of yin and yang in actual daily diet.

The following types of women are apt to have hare-lipped children.

1. Those who urinate more than three times in 24 hours.
2. Exophthalmic women (protruding eyes).
3. Those who have an enlarged thyroid gland.
4. Those who have freckles.
5. Those who shed tears very easily.
6. Those who love fruit.
7. Those who eat melons, eggplant, and potatoes.
8. Those who like sweets.
9. Those who are sluggish and absent-minded and have poor memories.
10. Those whose faces are loose and very dark.

The woman who has more than three of these peculiarities has the greatest tendency to have a hare-lipped child.

One finds that a large number of hare-lipped babies are conceived during August and September. Why? Because around this period, foods which have the power to disjoin, to separate (yin foods with a potassium/sodium ratio of more than 5:1) are produced and sold in large quantities. Pregnant women unsuspectingly eat them with delight.

As a rule, when a woman conceives in the month of July or August and, in addition, has characteristics 1, 6, 7 and 8, she will bear a child with a large mouth or a hare-lip. But even the woman who conceives in November or December who continually eats oranges, apples, melons or other fruits, eggplant or potatoes, brings a hare-lipped infant into the world.

The Seven Stages of Judgment

Our happiness depends upon our judgment. Illness or health, intelligence or foolishness, piety or vice depend upon our judgment. Judgment develops upward toward perfection, in the way I show below, from one to seven.

1. Physical judgment (mechanical and blind judgment).
2. Sensorial judgment (pleasant and unpleasant).
3. Sentimental judgment (what is desirable and undesirable).
4. Conceptual judgment (intellectual, scientific).
5. Social judgment (social reason's judgment: morals and economy).
6. Judgment of thought and thinking power (justice and injustice).
7. Absolute and universal love that embraces everything and turns every antagonism into complementarism.

At the time of birth and for some time thereafter, we are unable to form any judgment. Then the physical judgment, the lowest one, awakens.

After some days the sensorial judgment begins to function and to perceive cold and warmth, two poles of our relative world. It develops from day to day, and gradually can distinguish all the degrees between two extremes: colors, shapes, temperatures, agreeable or disagreeable tastes, sympathy or hostility. This latter stage of development occurs within a few weeks.

After some months, we reach the affective or sentimental judgment. We discern what attracts us and what frightens us or may harm us, etc.

In the fourth stage, judgment develops in us the true concept of the two antagonistic categories: good and evil, nice and ugly, useful and useless, healthy food and poison, just and unjust; as well as all natural or scientific categories.

On reaching the fifth stage, judgment turns social and perceives a wider horizon: economy and morality.

In the sixth stage, ideology develops (dualism, materialism, spiritualism, life's affirmation or negation, etc.)

It is in the seventh stage, the very last one, that our judging ability reaches the constitution of the universe and life, where we are able to embrace all opposites in order to establish the grand universal unification.

Such is, in my opinion, a general sketch of the natural development of our judgment. It is innate and can be likened to memory, the basis of our faculty for adaptation, and its expansion is but our self-realization (or the realization of life itself). This realization can be destroyed, deformed, and repressed under the influence of the biological, physiological and social surroundings during childhood. It is then the beginning of our misfortune and the reason why some souls are detained and remain behind.

Their judging remains childish and primitive. This is the case with all those who look toward symptomatic medicine, all those who love wealth, strength, and authority, such as famous politicians, industrialists, soldiers, and physicians. Of course, they are not entirely responsible for this state of mind; but their surroundings are greatly responsible, for they impede and stop the natural and total development of judgment.

Some people try to achieve the supreme judging ability by endeavoring to live like great men of history. But it is obvious that imitation is a mistake. Being very pious, may not these people also be very egoistic? If you are anxious to see what becomes of such people, visit India, the great Buddha's birthplace. There in the streets of Calcutta you will see a poor clerk giving a copper to a beggar, or a merchant placing one or several hundred annas (worth two cents each) at his shop entrance every morning for beggars. There are hundreds of thousands of beggars. As a matter of fact, there are in India many philanthropic millionaires and beggars because it is a part of professional religions. Poor officials or clerks distribute food every morning, year in and year out, to hundreds of beggars. This food is contributed by neighbors and by the rich. It is a social industry.

The Unique Principle teaches, "the nicer the front, the uglier the back." Such is the back of India, mother of great religions. Such is the end of a country that was established according to altruistic principles. But it is not to be forgotten that "the greater and wider the face, the greater and wider the back." This means that besides these so-called philanthropists, there are some who are really benefactors.

In any case, one cannot possess the supreme judging ability from the very beginning. One must first develop the lowest judgment. Therefore one must endure heat, cold, hunger and the greatest difficulties, not only in childhood, but all during one's entire life. And as one grows older, life seems more agitated and full of difficulties and sadness. One must love and be betrayed.

Without having lived such a life, one cannot and must not unfold one's conceptual faculty of judgment. Later, the judging ability expands, through social and ideological life to the supreme ability. And the supreme judging ability must be strengthened, developed and increased infinitely by training the lower categories of judgment at the same time as the higher ones, since "the greater and wider the back, the greater and wider the front." The seven stages of judgment are not alien to and independent of each other, but just different degrees of the same judging ability. They are the roots, trunk, boughs, foliage, flowers and fruit of this 'judgment tree.' In order for boughs to develop and for flowers and fruit to be produced in large quantities under a fine sky, there must be thick and thin roots reaching deep into rich black soil.

The Order of the Universe and the Unique Principle

The Order of the Universe is governed by seven principles which constitute the universal logic.

1. What has a beginning has an end.
2. All which has a front has a back.
3. There is nothing identical.
4. The bigger the front, the bigger the back.
5. All antagonism is complementary.
6. Yin and yang are the classifications of all polarization. They are antagonistic and complementary.
7. Yin and yang are the two arms of the One (Infinity).

These principles are, first of all, dynamic; that is why they are opposite to formal logic, which is static. They can be applied to any domain, at any level of life, and to all things existing in the universe of relativity. Moreover, they can unify all antagonisms.

Formal logic is rigid; it is a simple snapshot of life in the infinite universe, thus, infinitesimally analytical without intending or knowing; whereas universal logic is a living image of all life and all things. Formal logic destroys continuity: the principle of identity, the principle of contradiction, the principle of exclusive environments, shows us only a static, finite image, an image imprisoned in the static world, determined from appearance, built on our senses or our instruments. In reality, all things in this world change, without ceasing, from one extreme to the other. Nothing is stable or constant in this relative world. Those who do not see this fact look for constants.

And everything they think to be constant is only an instantaneous "snap" — illusory, non-living, and infinitesimal — of the infinite and eternal universe. Analytical eyes are blind in the infinite universe.

*   *   *

The seven principles of the Order of the Universe are completed by the twelve theorems of the Unique Principle: yin and yang. These theorems define the functioning of the world of relativity.

1. Yin and yang are the two poles of infinite pure expansion.
2. Yin and yang are produced continually by the infinite expansion.
3. Yin is centrifugal (expansive); yang is centripetal (contractive). Yin and yang produce energy.
4. Yin attracts yang and yang attracts yin.
5. Yin and yang, combined in variable proportions, produce all phenomena.
6. All phenomena are constantly changing their yin and yang components. Everything is without rest.
7. Nothing is totally yin nor totally yang; all is relative.
8. Nothing is neuter. Yin or yang is in excess in every case.
9. The force of attraction is proportional to the difference of the components of yin and yang.
10. Yin repels yin and yang repels yang. The greater the difference, the weaker the repulsion.
11. With time and space, yin produces yang and yang produces yin.
12. Everything is yang at its center and yin at its surface.

Reference Notes

1 For further explanation of the Unique Principle, see "The Order of the Universe and the Unique Principle," page 124.

2 For recipes, see *The Do of Cooking* by Cornellia Aihara (G.O.M.F. Press, 1982) and *The First Macrobiotic Cookbook* (G.O.M.F. Press, 1984).

3 This is an example of how to apply the Unique Principle in medicine; burnt carbon (extreme yang) is used to treat a yin condition. — H.A.

4 It is traditional in Japan for a pregnant woman to wear a wide cotton sash (*obi*) tied firmly around the abdomen to support the organs and to prevent the baby from growing too quickly, thus ensuring an easy delivery. — H.A.

5 For recipes, see *The Calendar Cookbook* by Cornellia Aihara (G.O.M.F. Press, 1979).

6 For recipe, see *The Calendar Cookbook* by Cornellia Aihara (G.O.M.F. Press, 1979).

7 For recipes, see *The First Macrobiotic Cookbook* (G.O.M.F. Press, 1984).

8 Recent studies confirm this. For further discussion of milk in human diet, see *Don't Drink Your Milk!* by Frank Oski, M.D., Mollica Press, Syracuse, New York, 1983, and *Milk, A Myth of Civilization* by Herman Aihara, Grain & Salt Society, Magalia, California, 1983.

9 Ohsawa was writing at the beginning of Japan's involvement with World War II, in 1941; what he predicted in fact came to pass. —H.A.

10 *Haiku* is a Japanese verse form consisting of exactly seventeen syllables. Each *haiku* offers a glimpse of nature itself, at a specific place and season, but without any expression of human emotion. —H.A.

11 For further discussion, see "The Seven Stages of Judgment," page 121.

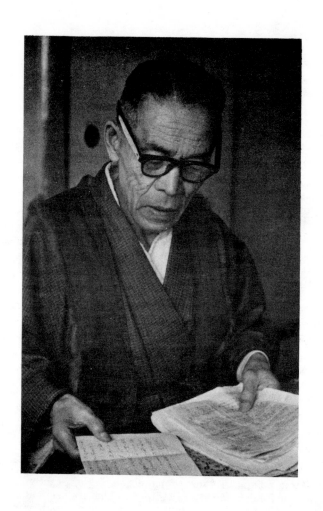

About the Author

George Ohsawa (Yukikazu Sakurazawa) was born in Kyoto, the old capital of Japan, on October 18, 1893.

He is the author of over three hundred books, ten of which have been published in France since 1926. His work *A New Theory of Nutrition and Its Therapeutic Effect*, written and published in Japan in 1920, is in its seven hundredth edition.

Thirty years of his life were spent introducing Oriental culture to Europe, while simultaneously interpreting the culture of the West for Japan. Among his many tanslations into Japanese are *Man, the Unknown* by Alexis Carrel and *The Meeting of East and West* by F. S. C. Northrup.

His passing on April 24, 1966 deeply saddened the countless individuals who are eternally indebted to him for having given to them of Life itself. Their infinite gratitude is expressed in a continuation of the vital work he undertook and so ably pursued for over fifty-four years.

Other books by George Ohsawa
available from G.O.M.F. Press

The Book of Judgment

"...But I Love Fruits" (*with Neven Henaff*)

Jack and Mitie

Macrobiotics:
An Invitation to Health and Happiness

Macrobiotics: The Way of Healing
(originally *Cancer and the Philosophy of the Far East*)

You Are All Sanpaku

Zen Macrobiotics